The Ultimate Guide to Well Being

I0223731

The Ultimate Guide to Well Being

Achieving 100% Mental Well Being

By Jason Pegler

Jason Pegler

Published by:
Chipmunkapublishing's
PO Box 6872
Brentwood
Essex
CM13 1ZT
United Kingdom

http://www.chipmunkapublishing.com

The Ultimate Guide to Well Being

CONTENTS

Jason Pegler

ACKNOWLEDGEMENTS

I would like to dedicate this book to anybody who strives to help the well being of other people on the planet. I would also like to thank anyone who has been associated with Chipmunkapublishing and the Chipmunka Foundation over the last five years. Thank you for giving me the strength and support when I needed it most. In particular I would like to thank Andrew Latchford who is without doubt the most generous, patient and giving business partner, human being and friend that anyone could ever wish for. I would also like to thank Paul Williams, Paul Brandwood, Barbara Phillips, Mark Randall, John Bird, Nigel Kershaw, Ashley Cooke, Barbara Brown, Peter Horn, Charles Beckett, Stuart Bell, Sandra Lawman, Dominic O'Donnell, Ben Robertson, Nigel Stoneman, Former Labour MP and Cabinet Minister Tony Benn, Adele Blakebrough, Robert Bond, Dolly Sen, Dominic Hiatt. Apologies if I have not mentioned you.

I would also like to thank all the Chipmunkapublishing authors for believing that they and we can make a difference. Thank you for believing in me, and the Chipmunka team.

I would like to thank the many Chpimunka volunteers around the world for their time, donations, kindness and dedication in helping us to help more people. They can see that the work we are doing is a unique empowerment model that is changing the history of the mental health movement for the better.

I would like to give special thanks to the fifty or so university students around the world who have given their time to come into Chipmunka offices to selflessly help other people whose lives need to be given a voice. I would like to give a special thanks to students from French universities and London universities for giving up a considerable amount of their time and using their initiative to help more people.

There have been many organizations and people that have helped inspire me along the way. I would like to thank Virgin, My Space, You Tube, Microsoft, eBay, Apple, Manchester United, Anthony Robbins, Coldplay, Eminem, Dr Dre, Snoop Doggy Dogg, Paul McKenna, The Department of Trade & Industry, Bill Clinton, Tony Blair, Nelson Mandela, Bob Geldof, U2, David Beckham, Madonna, Ronnie O'Sullivan, Steven Spielberg, Martin Scorsese, Ben Affleck, Matt Damon, Al Pacino, Tom Cruise, Robert de Niro, Bill Gates, Paul Merton and Richard Branson, to name but a few.

I would like to thank particular organizations that do not always get the high profile but have an important role in the well being of people in the UK especially and further a field. Please forgive me for any organizations that have not been mentioned. You know who you are. I would like to whole heartedly thank the DTI, New Statesman, The Arts Council, The National Lottery, SLAM NHS Trust, NIMHE, London Development Centre, The Sunday Times, BBC, ITV, Channel 4, Sky TV, Big Issue, Community Action Network, Mind, Rethink, Sane, the Independent, Daily Telegraph, Guardian, The Times, The Observer, Natmags, Emap, Launchpad, KPMG, Faegre Benson Hobson & Audley, Olswang, CCHR, Samaritans, NAMHE,

I would like to thank my family and friends for allowing me to express the way I feel about the world during our time together. Thank you from the bottom of my heart. I would like to thank my partner Sonia for her love everyday that gives me the strength to continue the utopian dream that I have to eliminate the humiliation that people with 'mental health issues' feel or will ever feel and to make suicides a thing of the past. Your love, patience, kindness and advice inspire me everyday.

Jason Pegler

The Ultimate Guide to Well Being

Chapter One

Healthy, mind, body and soul

To discover the ultimate path to well being, you have to reach inside of your mind, body and soul like you never have before. This takes a conscious effort or *massive action* as Anthony Robbins most aptly calls it. Anthony Robbins who is probably regarded as the greatest motivational speaker on the planet says that you need to take *massive action* in his book Unlimited Power (Published by Simon & Schuster 1989). In the last 10 years I have read several hundred self-help books and regard Unlimited Power as the best of them all, much better than his later books and audio material. He is also a pretty impressive speaker – I have listened to him for many an hour.

Anthony Robbins is exactly right. There is no point in procrastinating on doing something. You have to actually do it. You have to look inside of yourself and ask yourself who you are as a human being and what you are capable of. Then do it.

Once you discover who you are, you can then discover what you want and then start doing it. It really is as simple as that and not rocket science. Just decide to do something and then take massive action.

During this book I have decided to split the journey to Ultimate Well Being into nine manageable steps (It's like two Stephen Covey books in one and a bonus chapter– only joking, Steve, I am a big fan of your books Stephen … Please keep writing). Whilst you go through each step and go through each exercise, take notes, re read anything you do not understand and visualise the positive outcomes of each step so that you are also taking a step forward and are therefore a step closer to Ultimate Well Being. Each step will take you that little bit closer to 100% mental well being. See this book as an examination of yourself. You will be able to pass but you will have to challenge yourself to progress. This book is an opportunity for you to test yourself and give yourself 100% success, as you are the examiner of your life. Nobody else is responsible for how you feel… Just you… That is the reality. See this examination as a confirmation that you and anyone can choose to be a success and even rid yourself of your ego in the process so you can lead a more fulfilled life and have a more positive impact on the world. I repeat. You are the examiner in your life. Ultimately no matter where you seek inspiration the responsibility of living your life boils down to you and not anybody else.

This is not just another self-help book. Even if it were I do not think that would necessarily be a bad thing. I like self help books. They fill your head with positive things and day-to-day people can easily be bombarded with more negative than positive thoughts, so self-help can reprogramme positivism. My first two books document how I lived a life of manic-depression and cured myself. (If you feel this is dubious please break your pattern, open your mind, change your belief system, do whatever it takes to accept this as fact and then read on!) I have been in the depths of despair and welcomed positivism and enlightenment into my life and made the permanent switch into having a happy mind, body and soul. Therefore I feel that I am qualified to write a new type of self-help book and publish a new type of self-help genre of autobiographical memoirs from people who suffer 'mental illness'. I have changed my life and I am not just using some kind of theoretical system like most other self help books. My personal suffering has been revealed in my earlier books and the weaknesses of many self help writers is a mystery. Reading this book is a unique opportunity for you to totally enhance your life and reach new standards in every aspect of your life so you can be totally empowered.

You will be able to be a *novus homo* as they say in Latin. A new man as the amazing Roman orator Cicero was in 63BC when he became a member of the Equestrian Order through his achievements instead of through birth. Nobody had done that previously in the history of Rome so it really was an outstanding achievement. If you find it hard to identify with the life of someone over 2000 years ago in another city then think of rap.

Think of Eminem's lyrics in the film *8 Mile*. The director of *8 Mile* said that writing the lyrics for the film made Eminem go deeper inside himself than at any other time in his life. As Eminem says in the most famous track he wrote for the movie "*If you had one chance, one opportunity in life… would you capture it or let it slip*". In 8 Mile Eminem wins a rapping contest but instead of celebrating who goes back to work so he can save up money for his studio time. The implication in Eminem's lyrics I believe are that you should capture an opportunity even if you only have it once. This is exactly what Eminem does in the film and exactly why he won the contest and went back to work to save up for his studio time so Rabbit would become a famous rapper just like Eminem is.

Would you capture it or let it slip?

I remember being inspired when watching *8 Mile* and was fortunate that when an opportunity came along for me to make a rap album I managed to capture it and not let it slip. I have recently launched this rap album. Although it was a very steep learning curve over a short period of time and a lot of hard work, it was really much easier than I thought. The album is called *A Can of Madness*, the same name of my book and autobiography on living with manic-depression, published in 2002 by Chipmunkapublishing. I had one chance to do a rap album and took it. It all started when a volunteer in the Chipmunka office called Ama was reading the rap I wrote in *A Can of Madness* and said that she liked it and that she had a friend whose boyfriend was a rapper. I've always loved hip-hop ever since I heard NWA's 'Straight Outta Compton' at the age of 12. I see hip-hop as a potential force for good to bring cultures together and stop racism globally. I liked writing lyrics but never really thought of doing an album or performing. Soon enough I met Ama's friend and the rapper. His name was Ryan and at 17 years of age he had his own label, Raskil Records. I was amazed how good the rappers were on his label, especially as most of them were teenagers and they wanted to help people with mental illness. So within 6 weeks I had paid for and organised two rap events for them to perform live for the very first time. At the first event one of my friends whose rap name is Howling came along. He was a multi-talented 23 year-old at the time, and introduced me to his friend Avarice who made his beats. Avarice is a brilliant producer, lyricist and rapper himself and went out of his way to help. We held several sessions after work in my office and Avarice had given me a crash course in rapping in time to the beats to the lyrics that I had written a few years earlier. This consisted of several evening sessions after work in Chipmunka's main offices in central London. Then we spent one day round his house as he has his own studio and within four months of meeting him, I had launched my rap album.

Just like Eminem you can do anything like making a rap album if you wanted to. It's just a little example of how if you have a good feeling for something, that you should just go for it and reap the rewards whether they are emotional, financial, psychological or spiritual. In return I wanted to help Avarice, so I kept in touch and I am helping to promote his crew Renegade Artistry. Check them out at www.rarecords.net. They really are some of the most talented rappers in British Hip Hop.

Moment of Decision

As Anthony Robbins tells us it is in the moment of our decision when our lives change or we have a *paradigm shift* as Stephen Covey calls it. Anyone who hears and connects with Eminem in the film *8 Mile* could think of something in their lives that they have been hesitant about and would choose to go for it. If you read this book with this positive mentality and decisiveness then you will achieve Ultimate Well Being.

So congratulations to you dear readers for taking that quantum leap (Yes VISUALISE IT RIGHT NOW... feel good... that's not good enough... feel great... feel fantastic... that's more like it!!!) into a happier state of consciousness... OK... THEN LET'S PROCEED...

The Ultimate Guide to Well Being

We get what we focus on in life. In order to have a healthy mind, body and soul you need to treat these conditions as achievable qualities. Everyone has them so if you don't feel it stop moping around and just zap yourself with some amazing, fantastic, energising sense of feeling great for yourself, other people and the world as a whole. If someone tells you that you have manic depression and a chemical imbalance in the brain, they do not know what they are talking about. You can alter your chemistry by getting more oxygen and jogging in the morning. No psychiatrist has ever proven that there is something wrong with your brain so snap out of believing those negative thoughts. Life is worth living. Take it from me, I know! I have been so low I was suicidal for months at a time and I chose life. If *Forest Gump* can achieve the impossible then so can you my dear friend. And if you can… so can anyone…
So let's deconstruct having a healthy mind, body and soul into three parts. First, let's break them down into three separate parts. Then we will show how they are all connected.

Having a healthy mind.

Having a healthy mind is as achievable as you want it to be. Let's set some targets. Say out loud "my goal is to have a healthy mind body and soul 24 hours a day, seven days a week for the rest of my life." Feel good? Well good isn't good

enough… feel very good… feel outstanding…
Wooooooooooowwwwhhhhhh…… Great. Say it
again first in your mind. Then out loud. Now try
doing something fun with your body, like smiling,
while you are doing this or even be more
adventurous and try a flying kick… something to
give you more oxygen and change your
physiology so you are in a PEAK state…….
Repeat this three times… Feeling Great….. Now
CONTINUE.

Those of you who have been to an Anthony
Robbins Seminar will know exactly what I am
talking about. Don't worry if you haven't. Ever
seen Paul McKenna? Now you have re-
programmed your mind as Paul McKenna would
say to make this feeling of feeling GREAT a
reality. The more intensely you practice this
INCANTATION and awaken, the more real it will
become. Why not commit to chanting to your first
step to Ultimate Well Being three times a day for
the next year, after that it will be automatic. Now
you have programmed your mind to choose a
healthy mind you can mark yourself and give
yourself 1% towards Ultimate Well Being.

Congratulations, you only have 99% to go.
This will be as easy as you wish it to be. And you
will remember the decisions you have made in this
book forever because you are consciously
choosing to do so. Now celebrate as if your
favourite football team has just scored! Or for all
you ladies reading this, as if you have just bought

a beautiful outfit that you feel stunning in and the man or woman of your dreams walks straight up to you and asks you out. LOL... Or something else that will give you the same amazing feeling. Having just met your loved one for the first time! An end to world poverty... Every religion becoming friends... Something totally awesome and loving so you will NEVER FORGET THIS BEAUTIFUL MOMENT. Do whatever it takes to make this crucial moment in your personal development last forever and then multiply the love and intensity a MILLION TIMES. Close your eyes and have some beautiful intensity and love that will improve your life and the lives of those you love and even those that you haven't met forever. Feel the love and relax in a state of being.

Congratulations you are now fully on your way to ACHIEVING 100% and ULTIMATE WELL BEING. What's remarkable too is that this is a gift that you can pass on both consciously and unconsciously. You can pass this on so you can help other people and the world as one. Eckhart Tolle writes about this in *The Power of Now*. He is an amazing person. For the first 29 years of his life he was severely mentally ill. Then a profound spiritual transformation virtually dissolved his old identity and radically changed the course of his life. He did not know who he was, but spent three years on a spiritual high and lived for two years on a park bench in a state of ecstasy. The transition that transformed his life happened in a split second. Eckhart Tolle writes in his introduction in *The Power of Now* that he lived in a state of almost continuous anxiety interspersed with periods of suicidal depression. One night he woke up with absolute dread that was so intense, more intense than he had ever experienced. He had a deep loathing for everything in the world, his misery was compounded as he loathed himself more than anything else. During a time when he was going through the deepest psychological pain that he ever experienced, he broke through into a higher state of consciousness. Tolle writes:

"I cannot live with myself any longer." This was the thought that kept repeating itself in my mind. Then suddenly I became aware of what a peculiar thought it was. "Am I one or two? If I cannot live with myself, there must be two of me: the 'I' and the 'self' that 'I' cannot live with. "Maybe," I thought, "only one of them is real."

His massive action, paradigm step, step into Ultimate Well Being, step into being, personal transformation or whatever you want to call it, shows that anything is possible for a human being. Tolle is a living example that anyone's life no matter how desperate can improve.

The same is true of any kind of mental illness including manic-depression. I know this because I achieved the transition myself. When I was 17 I was diagnosed with manic-depression.

The Ultimate Guide to Well Being

From the ages 17-25 I spent over 1 year of my life in five different psychiatric hospitals. By the age of 29 I had made a 90% recovery but was still part of the medical system. In September 2005 I made a life changing decision after meeting Robbins whose work I'd been following. I used his techniques for inspiration in life and work for five years to take the final step to constant empowerment and Ultimate Well Being. I accepted that my manic-depression was entirely self-manifested and that I would come off the medication that was poisoning my mind and to come off it forever. I also managed to get sponsored by the NHS to go to his events, so that was a bonus and I felt justified in receiving this gift as my day job is as a social entrepreneur and learning his techniques would enable me to help more people anyway. Robbins and his techniques had helped but without being a social entrepreneur I would never had been able to make a full recovery. Both positive outcomes could be maximised to help even more people and give myself more personal growth and happiness.

There were 12,000 people hugging each other for four days. It was an uplifting experience that I will always cherish. Within four months of attending Robbins, I'd come off medication for good and had 25 people working for me full-time for free at my company Chipmunkapublishing's first office in London. This accelerated the utopian vision to change the way the world thinks about mental health and facilitated the launch of the Chipmunka Foundation (Registered charity number 1109537) and enabled me to help more people worldwide.

Every second of every day I looked inside my inner self, looking at what was truly important to me as a human being. As my mind became free of medication I became stronger every day and more fun to be around.

Within eight months of deciding to come off the medication, my life had totally changed. I spent three months coming off slowly with discussions with my psychiatrist who could see that I had massive insight into my own behaviour, life and belief systems and he gave me his full consent and support because he could see that I had total commitment with the intelligence, aptitude and mental strength to make a life changing commitment forever.

Now my psychiatrist is an active supporter in the active goals of my social enterprises and charity. How great is that? If you are a psychiatric patient this shows that you can totally cure yourself not just philosophically but in reality. It is just as easy as choosing to and following up with whatever you want to do in life.

By May 2005 I was sat in a room with 200 people at the Dali museum in London listening to the Channel 4 TV presenter Sarah Smith talking about how I had a vision for the world which shows massive potential for helping people cure themselves of mental illness, I was a phenomenal public speaker, extremely talented consultant, social entrepreneur who had written one of the most defining books of his generation etc... A few seconds later I was awarded the New Statesman's Young Social Entrepreneur of the year 2005, beating celebrity chef Jamie Oliver who has his own TV series and had convinced Tony Blair to commit to spending more money on every school dinner for pupils in schools throughout the country. All my dreams were starting to come true at a quicker pace because I had been setting the appropriate plans but also because I had chosen to take massive action myself and actually do it. I'd decided that it was only me who was responsible for what happened in my life. This is true for you too. If you want a healthy mind, body, soul or anything else in life then ultimately it is your responsibility to do something about it.

Now repeat after me: Me, myself and I choose to achieve 100% mental well being and I choose to do so now. Feel it, visualise it, imagine it, celebrate it...do it... Happy... Feeling great... Play your favourite song, shout it out, do it with a friend, meditate, play football or do martial arts while you are saying this to get more oxygen in your body... Do whatever it takes to make it have a stronger and more lasting impact on your newfound content and happy mind. Do this with your friend, partner, imaginary friend, remote control or any other inanimate object next to this book. Do it now, enjoy it and celebrate as if you have just won your favourite Olympic event and then donated your gold medal to charity for world peace... and say it five times so it stays with you.

Say that you will do it five times for the next five days and it will stay with you. Then every five days it becomes five times more intense and five times the fun. Who would not want that great felling to continue? Congratulations you can now give yourself 2% in your journey to 100% mental well-being and Ultimate Well Being.

Just like anyone else who is a PEAK PERFORMER, I constantly draw inspiration from people who have the greatest minds in history to challenge me everyday in my own mind and life so that I can help the people that The Chipmunka Group is designed to help. Some of my favourite inspirational figures in this world are:

1) Mohandas Gandhi (1869-1948). Known as Mahatma ('Great-Soul'), Gandhi was the leader of the Indian nationalist movement against British rule, and is widely considered the father of his country. His doctrine of non-violent protest to achieve political and social progress has been hugely influential.

Gandhi stuck to what he believed in. He had the peace of mind to continue non-violent and peaceful demonstrations despite being constantly pushed to the edge where most people have cracked under pressure and changed strategies even beginning to use violence. Gandhi stuck to his principles, made a bigger impact than using force would have done and went down in history as a force for social greatness.

2) From 1931 to 1948 Mother Teresa taught at St. Mary's High School in Calcutta, but the suffering and poverty she glimpsed outside the convent walls made such a deep impression on her that in 1948 she received permission from her superiors to leave the convent school and devote herself to working among the poorest of the poor in the slums of Calcutta. Although she had no funds, she depended on Divine Providence, and started an open-air school for slum children. Soon she was joined by voluntary helpers, and financial support was also forthcoming. This made it possible for her to extend the scope of her work.

On October 7, 1950, Mother Teresa received permission from the Holy See to start her own order, "The Missionaries of Charity", whose primary task was to love and care for those persons nobody was prepared to look after. In 1965 the Society became an International Religious Family by a decree of Pope Paul VI.

The Society of Missionaries has spread all over the world, including the former Soviet Union and Eastern European countries. They provide effective help to the poorest of the poor in a number of countries in Asia, Africa, and Latin America, and they undertake relief work in the wake of natural catastrophes such as floods, epidemics, famine, and for refugees. The order also has houses in North America, Europe and Australia, where they take care of the shut-ins, alcoholics, homeless, and AIDS sufferers. Mother Teresa is also someone whose mind I admire. She dedicated her life to helping other people less fortunate than herself. She goes down as number two in my list of most inspirational minds today.

3) I am also greatly inspired as many people are by the mind of Nelson Mandela. Nelson Mandela is one of the world's most revered statesmen, who led the struggle to replace the apartheid regime of South Africa with a multi-racial democracy.

Despite many years in jail, he emerged to become the country's first black president and to play a leading role in the drive for peace in other spheres of conflict. He won the Nobel Peace Prize in 1993.

Bob Geldof was right to call him the president of the world. Nelson Mandela gave his life to stop the suffering and discrimination felt by his people. He reaches my top ten minds today. My top minds may change on a daily basis as yours can, as there thousands of people that inspire me to push myself further and enable me to lead a more fulfilled, meaningful and loving life.

4) John Lennon also had an amazing mind. John Lennon's mind was so creative and he has given joy to millions of people. He created his own music and The Beatles are the most successful band in history. I like the way John Lennon went through stages and experimented with his mind. From songs such as 'Jealous Guy', 'All You Need is Love', his boyish humour and his peace demonstrations. His mind and his actions are truly inspirational to me.

5) Like many other people I have respect for Albert Einstein. Einstein changed the way we all think, by his theory of Relativity! I was never very good at Science at school but like many other people, I am inspired by Einstein's positive impact on the world. Einstein contributed more than any other scientist to the modern vision of physical reality. His special and general theories of relativity are still regarded as the most satisfactory model of the large-scale universe that we have.

(6) Pele was a genius on the football pitch. Pele was the greatest footballer of all time in many people's books, scoring over 1000 goals in his career. He stormed on the scene in the 1970 World Cup. He had a quick mind for football. He applied his mind to a higher standard than others

and was an amazing player to watch. By 1970 people thought that he was past it but he led Brazil to winning the world cup that year and was inspirational in the tournament. I am a big sports fan and watching the greats like Pele is one reason why I still enjoy playing football. I could quite easily come up with a list of 10 sportsmen who inspire me on a daily basis.

(7) I have always loved playing chess. Gary Kasparov makes my top ten minds of all time for today as he is probably the greatest chess player of all time. I know how demanding chess is mentally and physically as I played to a high competitive standard from the age of seven. Kasparov has won world titles and dominated the game for well over a decade. Kasparov is also an amazing person as he speaks articulately on human rights issues.

(8) Marcus Tallies Cicero - the famous Roman orator was a statesman, humanitarian and lawyer who was born 106BC- died 43BC. Cicero is one of my heroes of history. He rose from plebeian to statesman class, which was unprecedented and chose not to become a dictator in 60BC when asked to join the First Triumvirate, as he was not corrupted by political power. His philosophical work On Old Age is also the most sensible and helpful philosophical essay that I have ever read. It actually makes you look forward to old age.

9) Other minds that inspire me include William Shakespeare. Shakespeare wrote many amazing plays and beautiful sonnets which are still staged and known to people all over the world of all ages nearly 400 years after his death. His plays and poems move people through every single emotion: joy, fear, sorrow, pain, pleasure, humour, despair and enlightenment. Shakespeare's work touches every single facet of human emotion and has stood the test of time.

10) I also have a great deal of respect for Thomas Ssazz who has challenged psychiatry since the 1960s. Ssazz's writing has pioneered much service user thinking about psychiatry today and shown that the drug companies grip on the world of mental health patients worldwide need not last forever and can convince people to think in different ways.

I constantly use people throughout history to inspire me so I have a mindset that keeps me on my toes and raises my standards every second of every day. You can do the same. Write down the ten greatest minds that inspire you. Think of people who have changed the world or people who have had a profound impact on history, politics, sport, art, and literature. Even if it is your friends or family that inspire you most write their names down and then give reasons why.

Your top 10 minds

1
2
3
4
5
6
7
8
9
10

Finished your list now? That's great. You have now achieved 3% of your Ultimate Well Being. Write a line or two for each explaining how they inspire you to increase your score to 4%

1

2

The Ultimate Guide to Well Being

3

4

5

6

7

8

9

10

Now you have finished your list of people that inspire you and the reasons how they inspire read each person's name and the reasons out loud with passion in the same way you read out your incantation. Congratulations you have now achieved 5% mental well-being. Feeling good... ok.... FEELING GREAT......... that's better. I deliberately made the first few steps the most difficult. Now achieving your well being score should become easier as you go through the exercises.

NLP

The mind as you can see is an extremely powerful tool and so is the body. People who study NLP (Neuro-Linguistic Programming) realize now how important the way we use our bodies is. Fifty-five percent of how we communicate is through our physiology. Only 7% is from the words we use and 38% is from sound and tonality of the way we do things. Imagine you walk around standing upright, walking confidently and with an expression of calmness and friendliness. You will be able to send a positive vibe or give positive chi when you come into contact with people, if you maintain this positivism. You can even go further and deliberately be nice to people. This will have a positive impact on their day and yours. This is much better than walking and dragging your feet kicking, cussing, being cynical and placing your problems on other people etc... better stop there. I do not want to break your pattern and make you sad. Let's keep it up and positive. Happy... move on... Just a word of warning for you, don't be overly nice to people on an ongoing basis as this is not being honest with people. Better to be positive than negative though, as this is really important in your journey to Ultimate Well Being.

Think about the following. If you see someone walking down the road, looking angry, cursing and swearing, this will put your body in a different state... Your physiology will drop and somehow... turn negative... Your heart rate may increase... you may remember something that annoys you and your mood will drop as well... You may even cross the road... You may change the way you breathe or stop breathing... This could make you nervous... stressed... anxious.... give you a panic attack.... even give you Conversion Syndrome Disorder if you repeated this behaviour over a number of years...

See how the previous mindset triggered and caused this negativity.... It was self manifested.... You could do the exact opposite.... Think about it. You've already mastered your mind. You have the 10 greatest minds in history inspiring you and you know you can visualize more amazing people inspiring you in any walk of life at any moment to help you get to achieve whatever you want to in life……you can move forward at any moment when using your mind. You can do the same with your body too…

Walk down the road… smile… look at someone else and feel happy and smile… Your positive chi will pass onto the next person and so on… You will walk confidently… your physiology will be strong…. You will enjoy every second… look forward to what you are going to do and be happy in that present moment… and have a great day... This is something you chose and something that you decided to do.

I am now 31 years of age and my body is in better shape than it has ever been. I have more energy than I have ever had and average 6.30 hours sleep a day because that is all I require to have an amazing day each day. I believe that I am lucky to have a healthy body and look after it by eating healthy, exercising daily and not smoking. I believe that the healthier my body, the healthier and happier I am as a human being.

I know the positive impacts of a healthy lifestyle and playing football and or exercising most days, releases positive endorphins in my body that make me physically and therefore psychologically happier than I would have been without exercising.

The Ultimate Guide to Well Being

I still admire people in history who have the healthiest bodies of all time and step into their shoes to give me a psychological buzz at every opportunity I have consciously and unconsciously chosen to improve the condition of my body, which I know helps my related state, emotional well being and happiness.

Inspirational Bodies

(1) I have an amazing amount of respect for Lance Armstrong. Lance Armstrong won the Tour De France 6 times. The Tour De France is one of the most demanding physical challenges in any sporting event. No one else has won the Tour as many times as Lance Armstrong or as many times in a row. What makes the life of Lance Armstrong even more incredible is that he became ill with cancer, nearly died and still came back to win the Tour De France on his return. You think he did this by feeling sorry for himself... no way... he achieved this by deciding that he could overcome it and kept that positive mindset throughout.

(2) Second on my list of bodies that inspire me is Arnold Schwarzenegger. Arnold Schwarzenegger was born in a small town in Austria and became Mr. Universe 5 times. He trained unbelievably hard. When I used to play competitive rugby as a teenager it was Arnold Schwarzenegger who inspired me to go down to the gym even though I

had never met him. I knew no matter how many times I went to the gym that Arnold Schwarzenegger would look stronger than me. Imagining him as a potential opponent and imagining I was him when training inspired me to train more frequently and train harder. Rugby, like many sports is quite a psychological game and the stronger you look to your opponent, the stronger you feel and are makes a difference.

(3) Third in my list of remarkable bodies is Bruce Lee. He was renowned as the greatest martial artist in the world and was responsible for taking martial arts into Hollywood. In 1970 (Age 30): Bruce had injured his sacral nerve and experiences severe muscle spasms in his back while training. Doctors told him that he would never kick again. During the months of recovery he starts to document his training methods and his philosophy of Jeet Kune Do. Thirty years later this martial art is revered and practised all over the world and Bruce Lee inspires thousands of people to take up martial arts every year.

(4) Another body or person that I admire is Amir Khan. At 17 years of age he went to the Olympics and gained a sliver medal. Less than a year later he turned professional and beat the boxer who beat him in the final, has won his first ten professional fights and looks set to become a future World Boxing Champion.

(5) Houdini is the most famous magician of all time. Houdini is credited with the invention or unique improvement of a number of important illusions (the Strait Jacket Escape, Walking Through a Brick Wall, Metamorphosis, Buried Alive, the Hindu Needle Trick, the Chinese Water Torture Cell and the Milk Can Escape). He revolutionized magic and took it to another level. He could escape from things that other people could never have perceived before.

6) The most amazing magician and stunt performer David Blaine is also somebody who inspires me. David Blaine (4/04/1973 from Brooklyn, New York City) made his name as a performer of street and close-up magic. David Blaine has performed many stunts. For example in November 2000 Blaine began a stunt called "Frozen In Time". Blaine stood in a closet of ice, which was sculpted to fit his body, and a tube provided him with air and water while his urine was removed from another tube. He was encased in ice for 61 hours, 40 minutes and 15 seconds before being removed. Blaine survived as the whole world witnessed the event on television.

(7) I remember when I was 9 years old watching the Los Angeles Olympics on Television. Carl Lewis won the 100 metres, 200 metres, long jump and relay. On the biggest day of his life he

succeeded and was at the top of his sport for several years. All together he won 9 Olympic gold medals and 8 world championship gold medals. Although I never went on to enter the Olympics I found Carl Lewis an inspirational figure during and after that Olympics.

(8) Steven Redgrave is another amazing athlete. He is the only athlete in the history of the Olympics to win a gold medal in 5 different Olympics. Redgrave epitomizes the success that an individual can have at peak performance for the longest interval. He has also won the BBC's sports personality of the year.

9) Phil Taylor is someone who deserves a lot of admiration. He has fantastic eyesight and hand to eye coordination. Phil Taylor was born on 13/08/60 and is a multi word champion darts player, considered by most to be the greatest ever. His nickname is 'The Power'. Taylor has now clocked up 11 PDC World Championships to bring his haul to 13 world titles. Knowing how hard he practices I would not bet against him winning any more world titles.

10) Michael Jordan is another amazing athlete. He is the greatest basketball player of all time. He also made a comeback at the age of 35. Jordan put in the effort. He practiced before everyone else did for 1 year when his high school coach

refused to pick him. Next year he got in the team and the rest is history.

Now think of 10 people with the most amazing bodies in history that inspire you.

1
2
3
4
5
6
7
8
9
10

Great......Well Done...... Feel the rush...... Feel the buzz...... Coming up..... GETTING HIGHER. Feel that natural feeling of Ultimate Well Being......

Now you are 6% on your way to Ultimate Well Being. Write a line or two on why each one inspires you to get to 7%.

1

2

3

4

5

6

7

8

9

10

Read out loudly the names of the people whose bodies inspire you and why and you have 8% Ultimate Well Being. Congratulations. You are well on your way to leading a happier life....

Having a healthy Soul

Make sure you do not mention the same people in this section as you did in the healthy mind or body section. That would make it too easy…. Draw inspiration from different sources to maximize your well being.

Now you have a healthy mind and body why not go all the way and choose to have a healthy soul. There are many people throughout history who have a healthy soul.

(1) Top of my list today is Jesus. I was born a Christian but I am not particularly religious. I see myself more as a humanitarian with a mindset similar to some aspects of Buddhism. Like many people I see myself as someone who draws inspiration from everyone who has a positive impact on the world. I see my duty in life as a communicator of Ultimate Well Being and Mental Health Empowerment. Whatever your religious beliefs Jesus was an amazingly generous person. Two thousand years after he walked the earth, Jesus of Nazareth remains one of those most talked-about and influential people who had ever lived. Jesus dedicated his life to helping others and even died for us. How's that for having a beautiful soul.

(2) Martin Luther King also had an amazing soul. He was instrumental in giving black people a voice in America, reducing racism and giving equality to black people throughout the world. He died for what he believed in and has had a positive impact on the whole world.

(3)In my mind, Bill Gates has an amazing soul. He had a dream to give everyone in the world the opportunity to have their own computer. He has been the richest man in the world for the last decade but gives away a high percentage of his wealth for charitable causes.

(4) Dale Carnegie also has a beautiful soul. He was the wealthiest man in the world and was ruthless but then went back to a commitment that he made at the age of 30. By the time he would die, he promised to redistribute his wealth for the benefit of society and for the education of the world and he made sure he did. He accomplished so much, setting up schools and libraries that would not have been set up without his help.

(5) In my view Anthony Robbins, the world's leader in motivational seminars, also has a beautiful soul. He is driven by the will to encourage everyone he meets to reach their full potential in life.

Now come up with 5 souls in the world that you inspire. It can be famous people or people you know.

1
2
3
4
5

You know the score… Twenty Thousand hardcore knocking at your door… Only joking… Write a line or two on why each of them inspires you to take your well being score to 10%. Celebrate…. Jump up in the air… SMILE TO YOURSELF… however you want. Enjoy the natural rush and feeling of Ultimate Well Being.

1

2

3

4

5

When you have written this down and read it out loud and agree to at the utmost intensity like you have never meant anything before, you will have completed 11% of your journey to Ultimate Well Being.

As you have gone through each exercise, you may have been thinking of the same people for different categories. I know I did. I asked you not to repeat the same people to make your journey to ultimate well being more rewarding and more soul searching. I never said it was going to be easy but I promise you if you follow the techniques in this book verbatim and give everything that you've got, then you will be able to move forward and have the opportunity to make 100% ultimate well being a reality. There is no reason why you will not be able to keep that reality. This choice has already been made by you so congratulations once again…. you are well on your way to Ultimate Well Being.

You will see now that there are people who can fit into all these categories and people who do not for one reason or other. To achieve 100% mental well being you have to succeed in every category. Winston Churchill had a great mind. He was Prime minister, he had a great soul, he is said to have saved Britain in its hour of need. He didn't need much sleep. He was overweight, a drunk and a smoker and suffered from depression. In my eyes Churchill fails in one category, possibly two so realize how far you are going to stretch yourself. You are now only at 11% so there is a long way to go but you can choose to do it. Be like NIKE or somebody who inspires you- Just do it.

You can go further in your guide to Ultimate Well Being than Winston Churchill did, one of the most accomplished statesmen of the 20th Century. There is no reason why you can't be successful in all three categories. I have a healthy mind, body and soul because I have identified what constitutes having a healthy mind, body soul every day means for me.

When I worked out what having a healthy mind means to me I decided that it meant a mind free from medication, drugs and alcohol abuse. I choose to use my mind everyday to spend time doing what I am passionate about and learning more and more about philanthropy, social entrepreneurship, mental health, well being, business practices, social justice, information technology, Neuro-Linguistic Programming, the world and other things. I learnt to appreciate my friends and family more and appreciate simple things in life/ Live in the now and not worry so much about the past and the future.

I see life as a gift and I believe that I have an opportunity and duty to use the previous pain that I have experienced as a former manic depressive as a force for social good to have a positive impact on the world. I believe that I can facilitate changing the way the world thinks about mental health for the better and empower millions of people around the world to empower each other and give each other a voice so that in 50 years time there will be no humiliation for anyone who is regarded as "mentally ill". The moment that I realized I was in a mental institution at the age of 17, was the defining moment of my life. The first thought that went through my mind was that the humiliation I felt was unjust and I knew that when I chose to, I would spend the rest of my life finding a way to prevent other people going through the same humiliation that I felt.

I can say three things about having a healthy mind, body and soul.

1 My healthy mind is a crucial tool in reaching the most important personal goals in my life.

2 My healthy body is another helpful tool in achieving my personal happiness.

Chapter 2

Know what is crucial to your happiness

In the first chapter you learnt how to establish a healthy, mind, body and soul for the rest of your life. You realized that this was a choice that you made and attainable when you decided to do so.

In this chapter you will learn what is crucial to your happiness as a human being.

Think of your life and how hectic it is. There are many things that we plan to do in a day but do we ever get everything done? Of course not... Life would be boring if we did get everything done. That's not what life is about. Life is about, 'knowing thyself'- this old Greek adage is just as relevant today as it was 2500 years ago. To discover what you want to do in life, in business, relationships or relaxation, it helps to plan. However, this is not always the case. For example if you can be in a constant state of being then you may be able to move from one flow to another but this is not practical for most people to suddenly step into and is a complex line of thought. It is not in my nature to plan. I am by nature impulsive and have a stream of conscious style to my writing and thought processes. If something feels right then I tend to go with the flow that I have.

To get the most of your well being however and to know what is crucial to your happiness, it helps to plan, certainly until you move into higher states of consciousness and spirituality which are discussed in Chapter 6.

A pioneering exercise to do which is used in most self-help books is to write things down. At the beginning of this chapter we are going to use Anthony Robbins's technique that has been rehashed by hundreds of authors writing self-help books since. For our purposes in this instance Robbins's earliest work of (1989) is ideal.

In **Unlimited Power**, Robbins writes about us writing down our top 20 values in no particular order in order to take steps for us in finding out exactly who we are and what are therefore the most important things to us.

Spend 5 minutes writing down your most important values. I'll give you an example. For me values that immediately come to mind are –

Love, healthy mind body and soul, companionship, loyalty, friendship, honesty, integrity, compassion and hard work.

Once you have written them, put them in order of priority with number 1 as the most important to you; e.g.

The Ultimate Guide to Well Being

Honesty (1)
Healthy mind body and soul (2)
Love (3)
Compassion (5)
Integrity (4)
Friendship (7)
Hard work (6).

Your Values:

1
2
3
4
5
6
7

Do not forget to put them in order of priority. You should have at least 7 values.
Then write a paragraph for each of the top 5 and why they are important to you. This brainstorming exercise will start getting you in the mood to really answer the question once and for all. How will I know what is crucial to my happiness?
Use my example of Having a healthy mind, body and soul to help you.

Example:

Value 2 - Having a healthy mind, body and soul

I know what makes me happy. Having a healthy mind, body and soul are important to me so that I can make the most out of the love of my girlfriend, friends, family and people who I meet in life and want to help and want to empower and give a voice. With my healthy mind, body and soul in place and awareness of my values, I am able to focus on what drives me to have a positive impact on society.

Top 5 values with explanatory paragraph:

Value

1

2

3

4

5

Congratulations now you have added your top 7 values and explained why your top 5 values are the most important you can move from 20% ultimate well being to 25%.

The rest of this Chapter is an example of how I have answered what is crucial to my happiness as a human being. For me it is helping other people with mental illness that feeds my happiness and motivates my goals and actions in life. Whilst you are reading please think of answering this question for yourself. There will be a space for you to write your own notes at the end of the chapter.

DIAGRAM.   1
Economic.   Final Steps.

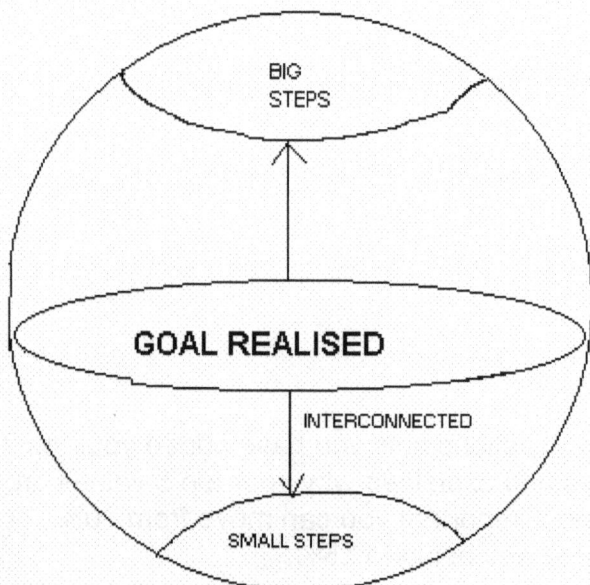

Non-economic.   First steps.

The diagram above illustrates how small and big steps can interconnect to realize a goal. This diagram can be used as a model to help you with your goals.

My main work goal in life is to reduce the humiliation of people with mental illness. I visualize this goal working so I can place it in the goal realized section in the diagram above. To achieve my goal I use a variety of steps. At the bottom of the diagram I put in the small steps. For example, in this section I would include the Chipmunka Foundation, the fact we help people with mental illness, the fact that I as an individual have had manic depression gives me credibility in working in this area.

In my view these steps are steps towards the goal. The big steps would be the Chipmunka Group, including Chipmunkapublishing. The fact that I set up Chipmunkapublishing as the Mental Health Publisher enabled me to set up the Chipmunka Foundation. Even if the Chipmunka Foundation achieves its mission and becomes the most effective mental health charity in the world it will not become a bigger influence than Chipmunkapublishing or the Chipmunka Group.

The Chipmunka Group is a social entrepreneurship and philanthropic model that enables the Foundation to grow organically. The Chipmunka Group generates its own revenue and actively supports the Foundation. It also gives opportunities to people with mental health issues to become self-employed, social entrepreneurs and show that people with mental health issues can achieve anything that they believe is possible therefore creating the world's first mental health celebrities.

The Chipmunka Group itself has the same mission as the Foundation but uses economic forces to take a bigger step. Therefore, all parts of the Chipmunka Group would go above the goal cylinder because of their economic potential in pushing the utopian agenda.

The fact that my life's mission is to help people with mental illness is also in my eyes a small step. By October 2006 Chipmunkapublishing alone receives more web traffic than any other mental health publisher on the Internet. This is because we are giving people a voice, an opportunity to have their voices heard in a world where they are discriminated against.

The reason why I have put helping people with mental illness as a small step is simple. I deliberately used the wrong language in the previous sentence and in diagram 2. There is no such thing as mental illness really. On one level it is a mindset. I know this because I spent 12 years blaming other people for my manic-depression. As soon as I stopped blaming others and took on full responsibility for my life on an ongoing basis I cured myself. It does not take a rocket scientist to work out that other people, such as Stephen Fry or Pete Doherty could do exactly the same thing. Mental illness can also be said quite rightly to be a manufactured term set up as a form of social control as governments do not generally want people to think for themselves. The term mental illness also fits the selfish entrepreneurial motives of drug companies to condemn and make money out of people taking medication that they profit from. On one level everyone in the world could be said to have a mental illness. On another level there are people who are suffering who need help and society should be able to help them. This could be a real dilemma without an appropriate solution.

The big step in the diagram and the solution is to improve the well being of people on the planet. The real voice here is changing the term mental illness and turning it into well being. If people see the issue as well being there will be no taboo and they will realize that mental illness affects everyone. Then they will be more inclined to talk about mental health and then more likely to help a person with mental health issues when they see them and not ignore them or judge them unfairly. They may even befriend them, give them an opportunity to get employed or manage their own life or money or offer them appropriate support. When I put my publisher's head on, this is quite exciting as in theory it means that I could publish a book on anything as long as I can find an appropriate mental health hook on it. If any serious venture capitalists are reading this please do get in touch.

The other advantage of using well being is also the mindset of the person with the "mental health

Jason Pegler

issue." They will see their state as something that can be felt by more people or even anyone and will also focusing on recovery rather than illness… Where people focus is massively important as where people focus is where they usually end up in life.

Then they can see a way out, change their mindset and cure themselves. With this paradigm shift the drug companies' and psychiatrists' influence on the world will lessen, their grips will loosen, their roles will be redefined or replaced and a new form of well being will be developed creating a healthier and happier world.

The final small step I would like to discuss is the fact that as a former manic-depressive, I have credibility in the area of "reducing the humiliation of people with mental illness."

By the time I'd set up Chipmunkapublishing in April 2002 and launched "A Can of Madness", my autobiography on living with manic-depression, I knew that my story was an example of someone who was prepared to face up to what being diagnosed with a mental illness meant in the eyes of society. In fact what motivated me to write it apart from knowing it would stop me committing suicide was to stop the humiliation and suffering of another 17 year old with manic-depression.

The Ultimate Guide to Well Being

This is because I went through it first when I was 17 and it is only natural to want to stop someone else going through the same pain that you went through, especially when you feel the pain could have been avoided and part of it was unjust on some level. This is a natural human instinct. I am no different than any other human being. This is precisely why my own experience is a small step in the universe. Even though my experience planted the seeds for the Chipmunka Group and the Foundation and is my driving force for realising my goal to eliminate global humiliation, It is my passion that makes me get up buzzing every single day and commit to doing more. It is my passion, which shapes my belief systems and well being. I am only one person, but I have a goal for the world.

The goal I have is to stop the humiliation of anyone who has been told they have a mental illness because this is an ideal. It is something that in my eyes should not occur in the 21st Century or should have ever occurred in history. This is a utopian goal but one that I believe is possible. The big step here is a founding generation of people stepping out as others and I have done, using mental health as a positive, thus creating a paradigm shift. I envisage millions of people stepping up around the world and saying why the humiliation of mental illness is wrong. This like anything, only receives real credibility and revolutionary status if it is led and controlled by the "sufferers" themselves, by the people who went through it. Otherwise everyone would be invited to alcoholics anonymous to give an opinion as to why certain people drink. The goal is beyond my own ego; it's beyond the Chipmunka Group. It's about millions of people all around the world being brave enough to stand up for what they believe in as human beings and having the mental strength to give back and take on the responsibility of giving others an opportunity to empower themselves for the well being of the world and the planet. This is for all of our future and for the future well being of the planet, for our children and our children's children, for people in the 3rd world so they can empower themselves and improve their well being and the rest of their lives, so we live in a humanitarian world for world peace and so we can motivate ourselves as a race to save the environment, stop diseases etc…

DIAGRAM
2:

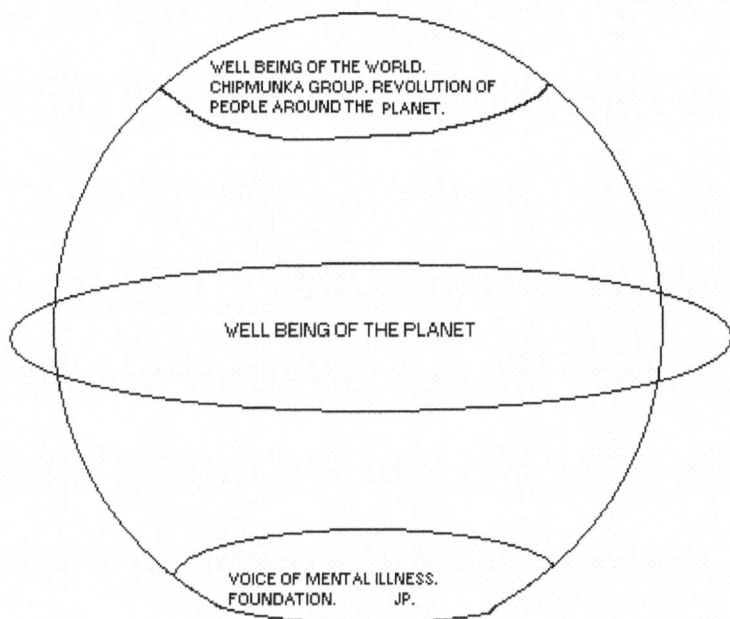

WELL BEING OF THE WORLD. CHIPMUNKA GROUP. REVOLUTION OF PEOPLE AROUND THE PLANET.

WELL BEING OF THE PLANET

VOICE OF MENTAL ILLNESS. FOUNDATION. JP.

This one goal that I have explained in the last few pages is an integral part of what makes me happy as a human being. I use the same thought processes in other aspects of my life as well. For example, the love of my partner, friends and family is also another crucial aspect to my happiness as a human being.

Think of something crucial in you life to your happiness. It could be in your relationships, work, health, finances, etc.

Now have a think about what is crucial to your happiness as a human being. No need to write it down. Just feel it and it will formulate in your unconscious mind.

YOU HAVE ALREADY ACHIEVED 25% towards Ultimate Well Being… take a few moments to congratulate yourself… pause… and enjoy the moment… visualize how great you will feel when you have finished this book and achieved 100% … feel good… feel great… YES… YES…This is called an incantation and is a technique you can use in any aspect of your life. Whenever you want to overcome an obstacle or stress or just want just want to enjoy the moment, you can always use an incantation to snap yourself into a positive mindset.

Chapter Three

Inspire Yourself

My healthy soul is equally, if not more important as how I act as a person determines my state of being and ultimate well being.

By being aware of having a healthy mind, body and soul I can be successful in having Ultimate Well Being and so can you.

Through becoming well trained in self-help, empowerment and Neuro-Linguistic Programming, I know that the healthier my body is the better equipped I am to fulfil my personal ambition of reducing the humiliation that anyone with a "mental health issue" faces. This is why I hardly touch alcohol or smoke or overeat. This is why I sleep as much as I need to and do not oversleep and why I eat healthily. I know that physical exercise gives me energy, so I work out most days. I regularly go jogging in the morning, play football every week, do weights, cardio vascular exercises and practice other sports including squash, swimming and martial arts.

I am also convinced that I have a happy soul. I am happy with my inner self because I have searched my soul and gone through a personal transformation where I consciously discovered what would make my soul happy and then lived by these rules that I set myself and I regularly review the guidelines I set myself. Therefore on an unconscious level my soul takes care of itself and is happy.

I know that the most important thing for my soul is to have a purpose in life that makes me a human being with a purpose. This makes me totally committed and happy in my relationships, has helped me find a peer group that I feel comfortable with and challenges me. For me it is important to have a peer group that is constantly growing and evolving. Otherwise I would lower my standards and get bored.

I am also totally convinced that the work that I do every day is a force for social good that other people around the world can benefit from today and in the future.

I set up Chipmunkapublishing, The Mental Health Publisher, to give a voice to other people diagnosed with mental illness around the world, so they too could join other people's goal of reducing stigma on mental health issues and my personal goal of stopping the humiliation that anyone with a mental illness feels and enable people to empower themselves through literature and multi media. This one thought alone is what gets me up with a spring in my step every day. This is why I work so hard and put my whole life into changing things. I do this out of choosing to do first and then a kind of necessity because I am fortunate that I have had the insight to realize what ingredients I need for having my healthy mind, body and soul.

The final exercise for this chapter is for you to work out what gives you the peace of mind to realize what a healthy mind, body and soul means to you. I want you to spend at least 15 minutes doing this exercise. Do it… and enjoy it…
Write down at least 5 situations in each category of amazing things…situations or events that would make you feel totally fulfilled as a human being if they happened or were happening in your life. Once you have written this down, prioritise them putting them in order of significance, then put time frames around them.

You can use them as your Ultimate Well Being action plan for the rest of the book. When you have completed this stage learn them verbatim and you will have leaped from 11% to 20% Ultimate Well Being. If you do not complete this whole exercise then you only stay at 11%. Then and only then move onto the second chapter. I have given you my own example to act as a template. The number at the end of each example below illustrates the order of priority I gave it at the time that I wrote it. This is a good exercise to try and can be repeated any time you want to refocus your healthy Mind, Body and soul techniques. Notice that the order I wrote them down was not necessarily the order of priority that I gave each action. The more you write down the more the exercise will help you. I have found this exercise to be a wonderful experience. Sometimes I have written down over 30 points for each and prioritised them which have lead to rapid improvements in each area.

Example:

Mind Page:

Visualize happy days every day 1
Do the work that I enjoy 2
Spend time with people who have compassion 5
Switch off work in the evenings during the week 7
Do not look at emails on a Sunday 3
Read and complete the reading of one new book a fortnight 6
Be in a state of being rather than visualisation and enforced NLP
Finish writing my 4th book mental health Empowerment ASAP.

Body Page:

Drink more water 6
Go jogging 3 times a week 4

The Ultimate Guide to Well Being

Play football every week 3
Eat fruit every day 5
Make love regularly 2
Have a stronger physiology 1

Soul Page:

Help people on a daily basis 1
Help someone I do not know once a month for one hour 6
Spend quality time with my girlfriend 2
See good in other people 4
look to empower others 3
stay close to my family 5

Complete Your Mind, Body and Soul techniques below:

Mind Page:

Body Page:

Soul Page:

If you have prioritised them then congratulations.
You can now move on, as you are now 20% of
you way towards Ultimate Well Being. Remember
you can do this exercise whenever you feel like re-
evaluating so you can maintain Ultimate Well
Being for your mind, body and soul.

Chapter Four

Inspire Yourself and have time for other people

People can draw inspiration from others of course, but to achieve Ultimate Well Being as with achieving anything else in life the responsibility lies with oneself. Mohammed Ali is a great example of this. Muhammad Ali (born Cassius Marcellus Clay, Jr. on January 17, 1942 is a retired African American boxer. In 1999, Ali was crowned "Sportsman of the Century" by Sports Illustrated. He is a three-time World Heavyweight Boxing Champion.

Most people who have heard of Mohammed Ali whether they know much about boxing or not, regard him as the greatest boxer of all time. This is not just because he was a great boxer but because he projected this image and always described himself as the greatest.

Mohammed Ali was so intent on winning that he constantly referred to himself as being the greatest to raise his self esteem and empower himself as a boxer. The fact that it became true cannot be said to be a coincidence. In essence it was Ali's sheer belief and mindset that he was the greatest that made him the greatest. The Rumble in the Jungle is a great example of how Ali the underdog inspired himself to victory.

The Rumble in the Jungle

Ali regained his title on October 30, 1974 by defeating champion George Foreman in their bizarre bout in Kinshasa, Zaire. Hyped as "The Rumble in the Jungle", the fight was promoted by Don King who had served time in prison for killing his partner.

Almost no one, not even Ali's long-time supporter Howard Cosell, gave the former champion a chance of winning. Analysts pointed out that Joe Frazier and Ken Norton had given Ali four tough battles in the ring and two of them while Foreman had destroyed both in the second round.

The fight turned into a political symbol – Ali was taken to represent black consciousness and the fight against white power, Foreman taken to represent US arrogance. Ali was massively popular in Zaire and it is said that the enthusiastic support of the crowd assisted him in his victory.

In the fight, Ali took advantage of the young champion's one weakness – staying power. Foreman had won 37 of his 40 fights by knockout, most within three rounds or less, with Foreman's eight previous fights not going past the second round. Ali saw an opportunity to outlast Foreman, and capitalized on it.

Commentators expected Ali to box Foreman at distance using his superior speed and footwork but, instead, during the second round Ali retreated to the ropes inviting Foreman to hit him, while sporadically counterpunching and verbally taunting the younger man. Ali's plan was to enrage Foreman and absorb his best blows in order to exhaust him mentally and physically. The champion threw hundreds of punches in seven rounds but with decreasing technique and effect. This was later termed the "Rope-A-Dope".

By the end of the eighth round Foreman was clearly flagging and Ali made his move, turning Foreman off the ropes and executing a beautiful combination for the knockout. Foreman failed to make the count, and Ali had regained the title.

Just as Mohammed Ali inspired himself you can inspire yourself too. I do not mean go out and punch somebody. Please don't do that. The determination of successful sportsmen in this case a great boxer can be a strong metaphor for inspiring people in life.

I am inspired in my life by many things. I am inspired by the people I meet, by the things I want to achieve, by the wonderful world, technology, humanity and advancement in art, education and science that I witness as a citizen on a daily basis. I am happy in my relationships. I surround myself by positive people. I do not overspend which is something that makes me feel secure. A lot of people do not manage their money and therefore have a low financial intelligence, which can lead to great unhappiness. There are many books that you can read on financial intelligence. I have read many similar books. The *Rich Dad Poor Dad* series are the best that I have come across. I highly recommend them.

I choose to do the kind of work that I am passionate about. I avoid doing things that stress me out unnecessarily and embrace things that make me grow spiritually, emotionally and intellectually. I am very aware of what makes me happy so I focus on doing the things that make me content and happy. This is not only common sense but a deliberate mindset that breaks the pattern of any negative thoughts so that they are not allowed to manifest themselves.

All of us should be able to focus on the positive things in life thus making our lives more fulfilled. Most people though, focus more on negative things on a daily basis than on the positive. There are many reasons to speculate as to why this is the case. Robbins would argue because people's standards are not high enough. Perhaps it is because society embraces people who fit in and do as they are told and conform.

One thing that I have noticed is that people feel a connection with people when they are depressed. If people assume the worst then they assume that they will not be disappointed. This is playing it safe but is also a disastrous philosophy in life as it makes people content with being average. Therefore people have low expectations and lead mundane and unconscious lives, as they never break out of their comfort zone. They become failures and then meet other people like them who do not achieve anything. They both feel a connection with each other as they are alike and the dreams they once had disappear and are left to recite as a whim when they are much older.

The same is true of mental illness too and as a former manic-depressive I was a classical example. When someone is depressed they create a negative image of themselves. If someone else, their best friend feels compassion for them when they are depressed they will be more likely to be open about being depressed again. This can be detrimental because the person who acts depressed is doing it to gain significance and connection with the other person. Therefore unconsciously they are more likely to want to feel depressed again in front of their friend as they will feel significance and connection and we all need these two sensations. They are part of the human experience. So when someone feels depressed they are actually getting leverage over other people. If one can go manic as well that's real leverage as you can find people to connect with and give you significance in different ways. I have illustrated these examples to show that you can cure yourself from a mental illness. I know this because I have done this myself. As soon as I made the permanent decision never to go back to this self manifested feeling of significance and connection through depression and mania, I took full responsibility for my life and stopped blaming other people and moaning about circumstances instead of getting on with life.

Hence in less than one page I have articulated the cure for mental illness on a global level. Robbins has proved this change in action can help thousands of people around the world. It should not be limited to people who have to pay to go to seminars but should be brought inside the NHS and inside mental hospitals so people can make themselves better instead of spending their lives zombified on medication. Notice I did not need to medicate myself or anyone else to actually make myself better. I did it myself. As long as people with mental illness are not stigmatised, can be empowered to have their voices heard and taught that it is actually a great thing to take responsibility for their own lives and take massive action then this is a full proof system that can be attached to health authorities and individuals around the world. This is the future of the mental health industry not the medication time that we witness in *One Flew over the Cuckoo's Nest.*

In my own work during the last six years I have seen people's lives totally change and turn around for the better because we at Chipmunkapublishing gave them an opportunity to have their voices heard, not feel alone and empower themselves. Just go to the Chipmunkapublishing website at www.chipmunkapublishing.com and you will find many of these people. You can read their testimonies and see how they are helping the well being of others.

It is no coincidence that the most successful people in history are not scared of failure. In fact they are usually the people that have failed the most times to achieve what they have achieved. Successful people are not paralysed by the thought of failure. They deal with it and move on. Look at Walt Disney. He is a classical example of somebody who didn't take no for an answer.

Walter Elias Disney – December 5, 1901 – December 15, 1966, was an American film producer, director, screenwriter, voice actor, animator and philanthropist. As the co-founder of Walt Disney Productions, Walt became one of the best-known motion picture producers in the world. The corporation he co founded with his brother Roy, now known as The Walt Disney Company, today has annual revenues of approximately 30 billion US dollars.

In 1922, he started a small company called Laugh-O-Grams, which began by selling short animated films to local companies in Kansas City. By the time Walt had started to create The Alice Comedies, the company went bankrupt. Even though the company ended, Walt did not give up, he packed up what he had of his Alice Comedies and decided to move to Hollywood to try and start a new business.

When Disney arrived in Los Angeles, he had 40 dollars in his pocket and an unfinished cartoon in his suitcase. Interestingly, he first wanted to break away from animation, thinking he could not compete with the studios in New York City. Disney said that his first ambition was to be a film director. He went to every studio in town looking for directing work; they all promptly turned him down.

Due to the lack of success in live-action film, Disney went back to animation. His first Hollywood cartoon studio was a garage in his Uncle Robert's house. Disney sent an unfinished print to New York distributor Margaret Wrinkler, who promptly wrote back to him. She wanted a distribution deal with Disney for more live-action/animated shorts based upon *Alice's Wonderland*.

Disney looked up to his brother Roy, who was recovering from tuberculosis in a Los Angeles veteran's hospital. Disney pleaded with his brother to help him with his struggling studio, saying that he could not keep his finances straight without him. Roy agreed and left the hospital with his brother. He never went back and never had a recurrence of tuberculosis. That was the beginning of the Disney Brother's Studio.

One of the main things to remember about the life of Walt Disney is that he wouldn't take no for an answer. Another thing that Walt Disney had and you should have if you want to inspire yourself to live the life you have dreamt of is to embrace fear. Yes for you to inspire yourself you have to embrace fear and choose life. Do not let fear hold you back or you will never reach your full potential. As Robert De Niro's directorial debut so aptly explains when De Niro the bus driver is talking to his son:

"The worst thing in the world is wasted talent"

Chaz Palminteri who plays Sonny the gangster also comes up with an interesting line. When asked whether he would rather be feared or loved he comes up with the interesting line. "If I had to choose which. I would rather be feared. As with fear comes respect".

Well that may be fine for people who want to follow a gangster. I am saying do the exact opposite. Embrace fear and move on from it. Don't ever let it hold you back.

Another quality you need to inspire yourself is to stay focused on what you want to do. A great example of this is Isaac Newton. Sir Isaac Newton 1643 – 1727. Isaac Newton was the greatest English mathematician of his generation. He laid the foundation for differential and integral calculus. His work on optics and gravitation make him one of the greatest scientists the world has known. He once said:

"If I have ever made any valuable discoveries, it has been owing more to patient attention, than to any other talent".
Isaac Newton

So if you know what you want in life and know what inspires you, make sure that you stay focused on it every day. A one-degree shift one day, made consistent over a long period of time could lead to massive changes. This could be applied to anything; work goals, dieting, training to run a marathon etc… You can't just decide to go and run a marathon. You have to prepare for it and make changes consistently in order to do this task as you would any other concrete task.

Another way to be inspired is to know yourself. You can know your mind, body and soul – remember what you learnt in chapter one. You can also
Know what is crucial to your happiness – remember what you learnt in chapter 2.

In order to really know yourself you need to take full responsibility for your own life, make your own judgements/decisions and do not live in the shadows of others. You need to know thyself.

Now read closely so you can do the following exercise. Think of all the things that inspire you and write them down. This could be anything. It could be a person, a place or a thing, a feeling. Let me give you an example.

1. The way the sun rises in the morning
2. The way tiger woods plays golf
3. The way single mums bring up children
4. The movies that Stephen Spielberg makes
5. Eminem performing on stage
6. Bob Geldof committed to helping people in Africa
7. Coldplay's music and the way they play live
8. The way Tony Blair delivers his public speaking

9. The way Bill Gates made computers widely available
10. People who want to help other people.

Now write your list of 10 things that inspire you.

1
2
3
4
5
6
7
8
9
10

Now take a look at what you have written. You will see that most of my examples mention people who are recognised for being particularly good at something. Many of them were famous people. That was deliberate. Isaac Newtown also said something rather insightful once:

"If I have seen further, it is by standing on the shoulders of giants"

This is an interesting concept. Inspirational people seek inspiration from other inspirational people. This is common sense. Do not hold yourself back. If someone else or something inspires you feel it and make it part of you. This does not mean you have to change your character. If you are a shy person you may not want to go around and tell everyone what inspires you, just keep it to yourself and feel it. If you want to tell the world or give some inspiration to someone who you feel needs help then do that too. Do not underestimate or be sceptical about feeling and therefore being inspirational. It is not a form of arrogance or even part of the manifested self or ego. The world is a beautiful place and the whole universe and everything in it is inspirational. This is a fact of life. How you live your life and how inspired and independent you are depends on how much you choose to feel comfortable about the inspirational world around you.

In my life I learnt the hard way not to take anything for granted. When I was diagnosed with manic-depression in 1993 after spending six months in a mental hospital I was only 18 years of age. Whilst it knocked the stuffing out of me it also taught me a lot about life in a very short amount of time. It made more sensitive as a human being, made me know that at some point when I was brave enough I would dedicate my life to stopping others going through the pain and humiliation myself. I also knew there and then, the moment when I came down from mania and realized I was in a psychiatric hospital and my life had changed forever that I knew I would ultimately have to take full responsibility for my life to inspire myself and be independent if I was ever going to make that horrific experience a force for good for me and society. The realization of what has happened was at the same time the most harrowing and beautiful moment of my life. I have taught myself to always see that moment as a beautiful moment and that poignant few seconds of my life planted the seeds for my life's work.

Many people have defining moments in their lives and it is more often than not how they deal with these moments that determine how their lives pan out. It is one of the great things about being a human being that life is unpredictable and we are given options to move in ways and experience things that we can not always predict. Of course the world can be an unfair place but most people can alter their own destiny. We have to believe that otherwise we become lazy as a species.

There are many techniques that can be used to train the mind. I have practiced dozens of techniques over the years. The most fun and the most helpful were the techniques I picked up from Anthony Robbins' more advanced seminars. I would do a daily success ritual that lasted for 5 minutes and set the tone for having a great day. After practicing this routine for a year I found that having a great day became automatic. I even found that if I tried to be negative in anyway, I couldn't because I had programmed my mind to be extremely happy. I suggest anyone who has any kind of mental illness and finds it a burden to practice their own positive reinforcement ritual every day for 12 months and they too will get the same results. My Daily Incantation ritual is mapped out below. After you have read it there is space to write your own.

Training the Mind

JP Example of Daily Incantation

1) Daily Success Conditioning Ritual

a)   Jump out of bed and do Power Move every day – Peak State
b) 2nd State – Close Eyes Vision Yourself
c)   Celebrate – jump up and down and anchor that with your physiology
d)   Say out loud with conviction your 'I am' statements and your belief statements

2) By 18/10/2008

Hollywood Film Director. Winner of Best Oscar at 33 years old. Famous screenwriter with Sonia. Mentally outstanding living in L.A. and Chelsea.

3) I AM

Jason Pegler

Full of joy
Outstanding
Focused
Inspired
A leader

BELIEFS

1) I am making the world a better place
2) I am the greatest
3) I love the world

I now give myself permission to move into this vision

Imagine having completed all your visions and incantations. How does it feel 1 year after completion 18/10/2008. It feels fantastic.

Practicing my daily incantations gave me great confidence, improved my well being, and enabled me to accomplish things and feelings of ultimate Well Being that I had not even really imagined before. You can feel the same sense of Well Being, just create your own ritual. I would recommend five minutes each morning in front of the mirror, before you even clean your teeth as then you will spring out of bed and into action and will set the positive tone for the rest of the day. This is the way Anthony Robbins and Stephen

The Ultimate Guide to Well Being

Covey recommend to do it and you will get the most out of it this way.

Your Daily Incantation

1) Daily Success Conditioning Ritual

a) Jump out of bed and do Power Move every day – Peak State – Your Power Move will be some physical activity that you repeat ten times to build up the oxygen in your body. Mine was a high front kick that I learnt when doing Taekwondo. If you are unsure what Power Move to do try raising both your hands in the air and celebrating by punching your fists in the air.

b) 2nd State – Close Eyes Vision Yourself – Now select two or three clear goals that you wish to achieve in the next two years and imagine how you feel after completion. Mine were winning an Oscar, being happy with my girlfriend and living in Chelsea and Los Angeles.

Goals:

c) Celebrate – jump up and down and anchor that with your physiology. This celebration should last for 5-10 seconds at least.

d) Say out loud with conviction your 'I am' statements and your belief statements - come up with 5 adjectives, each of them should be words that describe how great you feel and then 3 positive belief statements.

Above is what you are going to do each day.

2) Date – 1 Year after I have achieved my goals =

_____

Write Goals again and feel the sense of achievement here. No more than two lines, be specific:

3) I AM – list your 5 positive adjectives of how you feel below. Write alongside my examples:

Full of joy -
Outstanding -
Focused -
Inspired -
A leader -

Belief Statements - Write yours alongside mine:

1)   I am making the world a better place -
2)   I am the greatest -
3)   I love the world -

"I now give myself permission to move into this vision" – read this out loud and have your eyes close when you say this and imagine how great it feels to have achieved your goals. Write down your goals again below and then practicing feeling the sensation:

Goals:

Now you have learnt the daily incantation ritual, practice it every day. Once you have practiced it every day for a month, you can revaluate it. You might find your goals, beliefs and feelings even more focused and inspired.

For listing ten things that inspired you earlier in this chapter and creating your own incantation ritual your Ultimate Well Being Score has increased from 25%-40%. List 5 things that are inspirational in anyway to you at this moment in time to take your score up from 40% to 45%. I have given you 5 things that inspire me as an example.

Jason's example:
1 helping others
2 being creative
3 being true to myself
4 inspirational people around me
5 sporting heroes and applying their mindset and principles to my life

Jason Pegler

My Five Inspirational Things:

1
2
3
4
5

Chapter Five

Inspire others and become a social entrepreneur

Look at any successful social entrepreneur such as Martin Luther King, Nelson Mandela, and Bob Geldof. These people make things happen because they have self-belief/conviction that what they want is good for society and others follow. This can be on a grand scale or at your local community talking to a homeless person and buying them breakfast one morning every week and just listening to them without judging them.

I have dedicated my life to becoming a social entrepreneur and feel that my life has a purpose because of what I do everyday. I remember not long ago I saw a tramp shaking at 6.00 in the morning on my way to work and I wanted to help so instead of giving him money, buying him an unhealthy breakfast I gave him mine and some dietary advice, gave him advice on how to sell the big issue and probably most importantly listened to his story.

When I wrote my own autobiography on living with Manic-depression *A Can of Madness* I received a grant from the government to give copies to people who it may have helped. I gave 300 copies to people in drug and alcohol rehab centres, as I knew they might identify with what I went through and hoped it would help them. When I set up Chipmunkapublishing "The Mental Health Publisher" in April 2002 I did so because I wanted to help other people who had been affected by mental illness. I wanted to stop the humiliation that they felt for being diagnosed with a mental illness and feeling alienated and worthless by society.

In October 2002 we published our second book *The World Is Full of Laughter*, an autobiography on schizophrenia written by Dolly Sen. Dolly said that writing her book "started out as a suicide note and ended up a celebration of life". Furthermore she was actually inspired to write her own book by reading *A Can of Madness* and the fact that I published it and believed in Dolly inspired her to help other people. Dolly often says that I was the first person to believe in her. This I find extremely humbling and proud because in the last five years Dolly has helped hundreds of people around the world to express their creativity and given them a voice just as we through Chipmunkapublishing gave her a voice by publishing her book and encouraging her to be proud of who she is and what she can achieve.

As I grew Chipmunkapublishing, any skills I picked up and opportunities that came my way I wanted to pass on to Chipmunka authors so they could raise their own self esteem, improve their lives and give a voice and help more people who have been part of the mental health system for whatever reason. Five years later Chipmunka has signed up nearly 500 authors around the world and each of those authors has gone on to help other people. I call this the Chipmunka domino effect. It is part of our mental health empowerment model at Chipmunka.

Once somebody helps someone then the person that is helped often becomes stronger i.e. has a potential to do more good. When an author has their book published it may be the first time in their lives that anyone has taken their views seriously. When the author hears the news that they are going to publish their self-esteem is raised as they have something positive to focus on and they know that someone or something believes in them and believes that what they are saying is true and is actually how they feel justifiably about their condition whatever it may be.

The day of the book launch is a day of positive reinforcement. The author's family and friends will be there and they will see the author in a different light not just as someone who has had a mental illness that they cared for or didn't understand but someone who has taken a negative experience and turned it into a positive and has become a published author to help inspire other people with similar conditions and experiences. The day of the launch is also an opportunity for the author to give a talk about why they wrote the book. Therefore the author now has a new identity as a public speaker and often gives more talks as a result. Later on, the author might start getting paid to give talks as they have become an expert by experience instead of a service user or 'former mental health patient' who is not part of society.

With publication author's start to give talks to the media for the first time which can also raise their self esteem and profile giving them opportunities to write freelance articles, encourage them to write more books or find employment. I have also helped several authors receive grants so that they can promote themselves, their books and help more people. This is a win win situation as we are all working together to help the community and empower others. The stronger Chipmunka becomes and the stronger each author becomes the more people we can support, give a voice to and the more we can help society to empower people with mental health issues so mental illness becomes a thing of the past. This is a utopia that I will always strive for as it is something that I believe in and something which helps my own well being, and the more I do it the more I can help more and more people.

Mental Health Empowerment

Changing the Way the World Thinks about Mental health

Mental health empowerment is a mindset. That is all. It is a perception of the mind. I began writing this book after I had learnt all the techniques that Anthony Robbins teaches. Robbins first appeared on the motivational scene in 1989 as a 25-year-old writing the highly praised self-help book Unlimited Power. Seen by his supporters as the most inspirational man on the planet and by others as an opportunist or that massive American salesman and seen by cynics as the con artist who charges people £500 - £1000 to go to a four day seminar. I first came across Robbins in 2000 when I read his material and applied his NLP methods. He is in my opinion the most articulate, practical and accessible NLP practitioner on the planet. So why mention Tony Robbins in my own book on Ultimate Well Being when describing Mental Health Empowerment. Well, because Anthony Robbins's legacy is symptomatic of a new line of thought in the world of mental health.

People with mental health issues are becoming more responsible and are slowly being given greater responsibility by the world at large. This paradigm shift as Stephen Covey would describe it if he were to focus on this has been occurring year on year for thousands of years in

Jason Pegler

Western culture. The madman was always humiliated and excluded in Ancient literature in Greek Tragedy where the ultimate punishment for hubris by the gods was not murder or torture but insanity. Only in Victorian times mad people were sharing the same cells as murderers and hung because the stigma was so great. Psychiatry came along as a kind of false police service and started medicating people to control them as a form of social control and drug companies cleverly took advantage of this making hundreds of billions of pounds for their shareholders. Then NLP grew in the 70s along with the mental health survivor movement, which gained a greater identity in the twentieth century. There were interesting thinkers like RD Laing, mental health charities forming across the world and Madpride as a concept and movement had a kind of inner logic of "being proud to be mad" which in my view harps back to the old Greek adage of live thyself.

So all along the essence of mental health empowerment lies in people who are mentally ill, taking control of their own lives being responsible for them and giving back so that they can help more people. In 1992 at the age of 17, I was diagnosed with manic-depression. After several years of procrastinating and moving in and out of madness I made the decision to write my own autobiography on living with manic depression *A Can of Madness* to save my own sanity and help other people.

The Ultimate Guide to Well Being

When I set up Chipmunkapublishing in 2002 as The Mental Health Publisher I was fortunate enough to have an insight into Mental Health Empowerment for the 21st Century and beyond. As Chipmunkapublishing documents how a generation of people with mental illness feel about their own lives and publishes books by carers, mental health charities, related organisations, employers we are facilitating Mental Health Empowerment. My work is an example of work being done by millions of people around the globe in giving a voice to people with mental health issues and breaking down the stigma. This book is not an attempt to praise what I am doing; it is an exercise to put my pulse and therefore yours and other people's pulses into breaking down the biggest taboo of all - mental illness. This book also aims to focus you on the positive transition of the chipmunka phenomenon i.e. what I describe as Mental Health Empowerment.

You may have a question. I know I do. Why is mental illness the biggest taboo of all? We are all human beings and whatever our religious or spiritual beliefs, we all know why we are going to die. We all fear death and losing our mind. On a daily basis any one us could lose our sanity as life is full of ups and downs and human beings as much as we like to think we are, are not invincible. Madness is something that is fascinating in the eye of the observer because it is something that we are all interested in but do not want to get too close to. Hence, the reason for the stigma.

The tools for the mentally ill to cure themselves have always been there and they always will be. We are now in many ways in an absurd time of self analysing in history. We might as well all be in a Woody Allen movie. We are told by governments around the world that 1 in 4 of us will have a mental illness of some kind at some time in our lives. By 2020 the World health organisation tells us that suicide will be the second most common form of death. Is this a global epidemic or just to be expected when you look at what is actually happening.

Everyone in the world could be said to have some kind of mental illness but many of them would be unaware of it as the have more pressing concerns. They need to avoid starvation, fight disease etc... We all feel up and down on a daily basis. Some of us more than others of course but we all feel this sense of imperfection - inequality as human beings. The only ones of us who don't are in contradiction to those who are e.g. those who are actually in some kind of psychosis i.e. a manic person who thinks they are god.

As psychiatry comes up with more and more mental illnesses every year, more and more people are being described as mentally ill. If this kept continuing for hundreds of years then everyone in the world would be diagnosed with a mental illness. Wouldn't that be fantastic if I was the head of the biggest pharmaceutical company in the world or even a major shareholder...? Interesting... Do not see this as cynical... It is a fact.... eventually everyone in the world could be diagnosed and if you sold the drugs that treated people you would be quid's in...

I do not see drug companies and psychiatrists having a handle on things forever for several reasons. For one so many people are aware of alternative treatments CBT (Cognitive Behavioural Therapy), NLP (Neuro- Linguistic Programming) etc... and these techniques, if used correctly are more effective than medication and do not poison your mind and body, therefore they will be more common place. There is also a lot of money to be made by generations of entrepreneurs who are into NLP, improving diet, physical exercise, gym owners etc..., healthy fruit and drink owners, giving up smoking, drinking, Buddhist retreats, self help etc... This is a huge market and new types of products will produce thousands of millionaires and hundreds of billionaires over the next fifty years.

Also taking Chipmunkapublishing as an example - we are already documenting the way tens of thousands of people with mental health issues feel about how they have been treated. If we could publish in some way 10 million books or experiences over the next 50 years then that is quite a lot of evidence that says how people have been abused, how they feel, how they got better etc... It doesn't take a rocket scientist to work out that these people and millions of people around the world who have experienced what they have will and are standing up and empowering themselves around the globe. If you thought Martin Luther King and Gandhi were an inspiration then just think about the mentally ill. They have been the most isolated group of people in the world and now they are empowering themselves so they can help the rest of the world come to terms with their own mental illness.

Being mentally ill in the past myself made me more sensitive as a person, gave me more the potential for greater good and gave me a mental toughness and will to become a success and help people that was not identifiable in my psyche before. If you struggle in life and can get over something then this gives you the potential to do more. Everyone knows that. It's a common truth.

With the Internet at our disposal people can have a voice and people's lives can change and improve. We are a consumerist generation. People can dictate what they want. There does not have to be any brand loyalty because people can buy something cheaper, better, cooler somewhere else on the web but people become involved with helping people because they know that we want to make a real difference and give people a voice. I, as an author and a CEO am just an example to someone who was once not well and then decided to give a voice to himself and others to help society.

5 ways in which Chipmunka helps authors:

1)   Giving them an opportunity to have their voices heard by publishing their story
2)   Encouraging authors to speak to the media
3)   Helping authors to get their own fundraising to promote themselves and help others
4)   Giving authors an opportunity to do other things e.g. give talks, write freelance articles
5)   Encourage authors to become leaders in their own particular area of experience/expertise so that they can raise their own profile and help more people.

The way that I help others may be different to the way that you help other people as I help people through my own work i.e. the nature of my work is for a social cause. Yours may be more straightforward – having time to listen to people at work if they are upset, being good to your friends, supporting your family, donating to charity etc…

Think of 5 ways in which you help or can commit to helping other people and write a few words on each of how you help these people or how you are going to help these people.

1)

2)

3)

4)

5)

You get 1% for each reason and 1% for each explanation = 55% on your way to Ultimate Well Being.

Chapter Six

How can you make the world a better place?

Every day I make a conscious effort to make the world a better place in some way. This is why I dedicated my life to giving a voice to people with mental health issues around the world. I believe passionately that I am making a difference in some positive way and the feedback I receive from people who understand what I am doing inspires and encourages me to do even more.

It took me many years of thinking and doing to get to this stage of contentment, happiness and fulfilment. From the ages of 17-25 I was self-manifesting my manic-depression and causing a lot of pain to my family, friends, people I was in relationships with and people I came into contact with. From the ages of 25-29 I had improved a lot and was generally a good influence on people but I was still rebuilding my life to some degree and had moments of fear, disbelief and great concern.

Gradually after being focused on helping make the world a better place for so long I feel that the world or universe kind of helped me. My attitude, belief systems and ability to help others gained momentum and enabled me to be content with myself and my own life and my role within it.

Jason Pegler

We can all make the world a better place in many different ways; by believing in other people, looking after the environment, being a good neighbour, respecting others, fulfilling our potential, helping others etc…

I had very strong belief systems and did some very powerful visualisations over quite a few years where I envisaged making the world a better place. The strong visualisation techniques I used took me nearer to achieving what I wanted to achieve every day. Every moment I consciously took to find the good in others and meditated my way into finding more people who could do more good and help more people. Everything in my life approved in some way as I was focusing on these positives. The paradigm shift that occurred was remarkable. The same will happen to you too as you practise your daily incantations.

Write below in a page how you too can make the world a better place. You will not increase your well being score during this exercise although you will be learning a crucial technique to Ultimate Well Being. The happiness people in life are those that care about the Universe, the world around them and others. So in many ways, what you are writing below is the essence of ultimate Well Being therefore marinating your Well Being score. Whenever you doubt your Well Being think of helping others.

How Can I Make The World A Better Place?

Chapter Seven

Connecting Spiritually

After doing my visualisation techniques for two years my positive chi, as I like to call it, empowerment became automatic. I had gone through different phases and intensities of NLP for 4-5 years, which meant I was automatically happy even when I ceased practising NLP. I still had a sense of great contentment and fulfilment. This is true to this day and will carry on being true as I am fulfilled and content with the life that I lead. I have a state of equilibrium and balance that I had never had previously in my life and will remain in this zone of Ultimate Well Being.

There is not one particular moment when I realised that this had happened. I felt as if sometimes that I would try to be happy and then once my girlfriend asked me, "aren't you happy now?" And I thought about it for a moment – yes I was – so I didn't actually need to practise myself or use any techniques to be happy. This was so simple and I couldn't believe it but it was true, especially after I had probably read over 300 self-help books in the previous 10 years and then this breakthrough in consciousness and clarity of thought and contentment happened almost unwittingly. I just felt the feeling of happiness and accepted it. This is a very simple thing to actually do. It just takes a little bit of concentration, perhaps an alteration in breathing and then you find yourself at one with yourself and in a state of Ultimate Well Being. Even if you only have that feeling for a split second then see if you can get back to it. The more you practise the more you will realise that it is easily attainable. Clear your mind of everything i.e. what you are going to do, what chores you have for the day and just BE for a moment, slow down you breathing or breathe – you will be amazed how many people do not breathe. Then just focus on a feeling of contentment.

There are many meditation exercises you can do to heighten you awareness of this state and anyone can achieve this state of contentment if they just rid themselves of the irrational mind.

Once you find this feeling of contentment Ultimate Well Being – remember what it feels like, how you breathe, what your body posture is like etc… so you can get back to it at anytime when you need to. The better you can achieve this on a conscious level the easier it will happen on an unconscious level and the more that you will feel it.

Whatever you religious beliefs are, even if you have none you must have some spiritual connection with your soul, spirit, mind. Let your ego die. How many friends does the existential cynic have? Are they ever truly happy? I think not. I used to be like that. Just feel the positive energy and connect spiritually to yourself and others and your life path will be smoother and more content.

5 things that make you me connect spiritually

1)   Knowing that I am making the world a better place
2)   Knowing that I am not responsible for the mental health of others
3)   I am happy with what I do, who I am and how I feel
4)   Believing that most people are essentially good
5)   Seeing the world/universe as an amazing, awe-inspiring place.

Explanation for each – to follow

5 things that connect you spiritually

1)
2)
3)
4)
5)

The Ultimate Guide to Well Being

Your Ultimate Well Being score increases from 55–60%. After you have listed 5 things that connect you spiritually and then increases from 60-65% when you add your reasons below.

1)

2)

3)

4)

5)

Congratulations you are now well on your way to Ultimate Well Being. Celebrate and feel the great feeling. Feel the sensation and celebrate.

Chapter Eight

**Making the impossible possible –
visualisation/emotional intelligence,
perception, live your dreams.**

"I am always doing that which I can not do, in
order that I may learn how to do it."
Pablo Picasso

"Life moves pretty fast. If you don't stop and look
around once in a while you could miss it. Ferris
Bueller in *Ferris Buelller's Day Off*.

All of our lives can sometimes feel a bit like the
way Matthew Broderick describes life in the film
Ferris Bueller's Day Off. That is why in order to
live an enjoyable life, the way one perceives life is
extremely important.

Having high 'Emotional intelligence' is also
vital in maximising one's potential and leading a
fulfilled life. Daniel Goleman has written about
'Emotional Intelligence' in several self help books.
Emotional Intelligence is the ability to get on with
other people. The more easily one can
communicate positively with other people the
more positive and satisfactory one's life usually is.

Emotional Intelligence is completely
different to one's I.Q. If somebody is a genius it
doesn't mean that one is happy. In fact often,

people who are great thinkers are often tormented with extremely unhappy lives. Recognised as one of the greatest writers of all time Proust was ill for most of his life. Nietzsche, another great writer and thinker was also ill for large periods of his life. In fact many of the world's greatest thinkers; artists, writers and politician's were tormented by living unfulfilled and unhappy lives. We all know about the apparent synergy between genius and insanity.

It makes perfect sense when Goleman argues that high Emotional Intelligence is a far more favourable attribute than having an equally high I.Q.

People who have achieved remarkable things in life have a focus and always have amazing self-belief. They are not necessarily more intelligent than other people. They may have a higher emotional intelligence, as they may be able to connect with other people on a higher level than other people. One thing that is different between the highest achievers and other people though is that the perception of people who achieve amazing things is different than other people.

Remember the visualisation techniques we learnt earlier in this book. These visualisation techniques can be used in any aspect of your life to make the impossible possible. This kind of positive reinforcement belief as I like to call it is one thing that is apparent in any instance of somebody making the impossible possible.

Jason Pegler

In 1999 Manchester United won the treble. This had never been done before in British football and may never happen again. The Manchester United players who were part of that winning season often refer to their Semi Final with Arsenal as the turning point of that season. Manchester United was doing well in the league and still in the Champions League when they faced their main rivals, Arsenal. Manchester United had not won anything so far that season. United were down to ten men towards the end of the game when Arsenal was awarded a penalty. Dennis Bergkamp's penalty was miraculously saved by Peter Schmeichel. That moment gave all the Manchester United players a new lease of life. If Arsenal had scored that penalty they were moments away from winning the tie. Instead the game turned around and Ryan Giggs was to score one of the greatest FA Cup goals of all time weaving his way through the Arsenal defence and keeping Manchester United's treble dreams alive.

On July 20, 1969, Commander Neil Armstrong became the first man on   the moon. He said the historic words, "One small step for man, and one giant leap for mankind." A camera in the Lunar Module provided live television coverage as Neil Armstrong climbed down the ladder to the surface of the moon. Here man had made the impossible possible? How had they done this? Thousands of people should take some credit. Of course, every member of the Apollo 11 crew played a major role, as did the whole of NASA, scientists who had worked on space travel, funders who had donated money. The list could go on as so many people would have directly and indirectly made the event more likely to happen. Somebody's perception was also possibly different to everybody else's, however. In President Kennedy's speech to Congress, on May 25, 1961, he expressed a concern that the United States was falling behind the Soviet Union in technology and prestige. He challenged the nation to put a man on the moon before the end of the decade. Although Kennedy had passed away, his vision for putting a man on the moon had lived on.

Success in life is almost always a matter of perception. What one's outlook is in life is often where one ends up. If I wake up in the morning and I feel relaxed, look forward to the day, see the beautiful sky and enjoy being woken up by the wonderful birds singing I am going to have a better day than if I think. "Oh no I have so much work to do, woken up again by the noisy birds", focusing on the cold and clouds and wish I had taken the day off.

It is as if every day, even every moment we have a choice as to how we want to lead our lives. Some people get trapped in a negative cycle of thinking and end up doing nothing except self-manifesting their own problems, blaming others and feeling sorry for themselves. I know because I used to be like this a long time ago before I started using NLP and writing. The kind of people with these negative perceptions will never achieve the impossible as they actually believe that they cannot achieve most things. They are the kinds of people that bring other people down as it gives them a sense of significance and makes them feel better about themselves. They are people that have negative perceptions. Everybody knows someone like this. Well the less you hang around with people with those perceptions the more you will achieve.

You can break their pattern and try to help them but mostly you will fail, as they will be placing a burden on you. If you work with people who have very low expectations of themselves then the best way for you to help them is to create a positive force field around them so their negative sense of self disappears. You will need the ability to be able to switch off when you finish work for the day so you are not overwhelmed by their negative self esteem and negative impact on the environment around you. Be careful, as you will need amazing self-belief to ensure that you keep growing if you are supporting other people at work, in your home and social life. This includes your family and friends. You can only carry so many people on your back.

You can of course help other people change their perceptions of themselves, especially if their perception of themselves is unfair or unjust.

The Ultimate Guide to Well Being

Bob Geldof's work over the last twenty years is a great example of this.

Band Aid is a British and Irish charity super group founded in 1984 by Bob Geldof and Midge Ure in order to raise money for famine relief in Ethiopia by releasing a record *"Do They Know It's Christmas?"* for the Christmas market. The single became the Christmas number one on that release and on two subsequent releases. It was produced by Trevor Horn.

Bob Geldof, after watching a television news report by Michael Buerk from famine stricken Ethiopia, was so moved by the plight of starving children that he decided to try and raise money using his contacts in pop music. Geldof enlisted the help of Midge Ure from the group Ultravox to help produce a charity record. Midge Ure took Geldof's lyrics and created the melody and backing track for the record. Geldof called many of the most popular performers of the time, persuading them to give their time for free. His one criterion for selection was how famous they were in order to maximize sales of the record.

The recording studio gave Band Aid 24 hours free to record and mix the record on 25 November 1984. The recording took place between 11am and 7pm and was filmed to release as the pop video. The first track to be put down was drums by

Phil Collins including the memorable opening 'African Drum' beat. Tony Hadley of Spandau Ballet was the first to record his vocal while a section sung by Status Quo was deemed unusable and replaced with the Paul Weller/Sting/Glen Gregory section. Paul Young has admitted since in a documentary that he knew his opening lines were written for David Bowie who was not able to make the recording but made a contribution to the B-side. Boy George arrived last at 6pm after Geldof woke him up by phone to have him flown over from New York on Concorde to record his solo part.

The following morning Geldof appeared on the Radio 1 Breakfast Show to promote the record and promised that every penny would go to the cause. This led to a standoff with the British Government, which refused to waive the

VAT (tax) on the sales of the single. Geldof made the headlines by publicly standing up to Prime Minister Margaret Thatcher and, sensing the strength of public feeling, the government backed down and donated the tax back to the charity.

The record was released on 15 December and went straight to number 1 in the UK pop charts outselling all the other records in the chart put together. It became the fastest selling single of all time in the UK, selling a million in the first week alone. It stayed at Number 1 for five weeks, selling over 3 million copies and becoming easily the biggest selling single ever in the UK. (It has since been passed by Elton John's tribute to Diana, Princess of Wales, but it is likely to keep selling in different versions for many years to come.)

The Name *"Band Aid"* was chosen because it had a double meaning. At one level it means *a band of musicians getting together to offer aid* but, at another level, it is also an acknowledgement of the fact that such a gesture is like putting a sticking plaster on a gaping wound and does not address the full extent of the problem of world famine.

The charity set up to handle the money raised is called The Band Aid Trust. This project kick started Live Aid the following year which became a global phenomenon raising over ten times as much money as the original Band Aid single.

The group has been reformed on three occasions, each time from the most successful British and Irish pop music performers of the time to record the same song at the same time of year. Co-writer Midge Ure has commented that "Every generation should have its own version".

I remember watching Live Aid from my living room at my parents' house in Gloucester in 1985. I would have been 10 years old at the time. For me it was the most moving moment of the 1980's. It made me realize how privileged I was to have a roof over my head, to be able to eat three meals a day and not to have any fatal diseases. Live Aid made me realize that I was luckier than most of the world and that I should never take that for granted. As I grew up sometimes I did take things for granted and sometimes I did not. I like to think that I learnt a real lesson that day, however. That if somebody believes in making something good for somebody else then that is a great feeling that they should hold on to and if it is heartfelt and just then other people will want to assist in strengthening a force for good.

When I attempt to define Chipmunka and what it means to me, I often think of myself as that ten-year-old watching Live Aid. What if we could have the same impact as Live Aid did in the world of mental health? Couldn't we too make the whole world stand up and listen and make the world a better place? If the equality of the world's mental health improved then people would be better able to cope with inequality and therefore the world would be a more just place. My perception of being able to make a real difference in the world's mental health enables me to have a positive outlook on well being and makes me want to continue dedicating my life to changing other people's perception on mental health issues.

The Ultimate Guide to Well Being

Every day I receive an email, letter or phone call from somebody who says that our work at Chipmunka has really made a difference to their own life or the life of somebody very close to them, and each time I hear something as positive as this I feel like doubling my determination and capacity to help somebody else and empower or educate more people. My perception alters and I focus on the sensation of achieving more of the impossible, i.e. living in a world where there are no suicides and where there is no such thing as mental illness. Living in a world where everyone who has suffered mental ill health has gotten better and helped someone else overcome their problems. It is this attempt to achieve the impossible that motivates me to do more and inspires me to make a difference. This kind of empowerment has a positive impact on other people and they do the same. They start to help people too, and thus we have the domino effect. It is amazing how many people can be helped on a daily basis because of these types of positive belief systems.

You can do the same with your life. You can achieve the impossible. This is a choice that only you will make. You are ultimately responsible for how you feel. You cannot pass that responsibility onto somebody else. That is unfair and unjust as they have their own life to lead. You can choose to be an optimist or a pessimist. You can try and be clever and say that optimism stems from unconscious fear and pessimism stems from a lack of moral imagination but that is only being intellectual and that will not get you anywhere.

You can empower yourself and others by having an aptitude for Emotional Intelligence. This will get you half way there, but in order to make the impossible possible you have to take responsibility for your own life. You can visualise all you want but unless you feel a sense of justification for your actions i.e. a need for doing something possible, then you will not achieve it. How you perceive what you plan to do is of vital importance. You cannot set yourself a task and then alter your perception.

Many times I have daydreamed of being World Snooker Champion as I love snooker but I have never got anywhere near even being a professional snooker player. I am not good enough, but that doesn't bother me as I still love the game. When Ronnie O Sullivan was very young, approximately 5 years old, he met Steve Davis, the then world snooker champion with his father and said that one day, he too would become World Snooker Champion. Fifteen or so years later, Ronnie O Sullivan did become World Snooker Champion and retold this story. Ronnie O Sullivan deserved to be World Snooker Champion because he made it happen. Instead of daydreaming it like me he altered his perception and actually did it. Could you become World Snooker Champion too, or could I? Well that is unlikely as Ronnie O Sullivan and Steve Davis have natural ability that is far superior to most people who play snooker, but it is the combination of *physis* and *furor* as the Greeks say that makes a difference. That is natural ability and hard work. I do not get disheartened that I am not the World Snooker Champion as I love the sport and admire watching the best players at the game. I enjoy watching other people succeed and I am fascinated by trying to work out how they are so good at something that I only have an amateurish understanding of.

There have been occasions in my life when I have achieved the impossible and there will have been similar occasions in your life too. Write down five occasions in your life when you achieved something that at one moment in time you thought you would never be able to achieve and then list 5 reasons as to how you got there. No matter how small or big the achievement seems put it down. Look at my examples to help you.

1)   Having a steady relationship – fell in love with a beautiful woman
2)   Achieved Ultimate Well Being - Stopped focusing on feeling mentally ill
3)   Work for myself – Saw an opportunity and took advantage of it

4)   Won Young Social Entrepreneur of The Year 2005 – passionate about the work I do and other people noticed

5)   Finished my autobiography A Can of Madness – decided to do it and did it.

6)   Passed my driving test and drive regularly – practised and felt like I deserved to drive as much as other people

7)   Repaid debts – Planning, restraint and focused on positive repercussions.

8)   Had David Cameron mention me in one of his speeches – Just happened no explanation

9)   Won Gloucester Chess Congress ahead of 244 competitors – practised, enjoyed the game and concentrated on winning each game, one at a time.

10)   Encourage other people to improve their mental health – Focused on my own model of helping myself and looked at ways other people could maximise their potential through techniques and opportunities that I used.

Your Top Ten examples of achieving the impossible;

1)

2)

3)

4)

5)

6)

7)

8)

9)

10)

For each of your ten examples no matter how big or small and each reason you will receive one percent well being. This will take your percentage from 65% at the end of the previous chapter to 85%. Congratulations you are 85% of your way towards Ultimate Well Being. Jump up and down and celebrate... Go wild...And praise yourself. The world is a fantastic place... Just feel these senses of Ultimate Well Being for a few moments.... and a few moments longer...

Now turn the page and read the final chapter to graduate to 100% ultimate well being.

Chapter Nine

Being Creative

"I'm always thinking about creating. My future starts when I wake up every morning. Every day I find something creative to do with my life."
Miles Davis

"There are two ways of being creative. One can sing and dance. Or one can create an environment in which singers and dancers flourish."
Warren G. Bennis

"Creativity is inventing, experimenting, growing, taking risks, breaking rules, making mistakes, and having fun."
Mary Lou Cook

Being creative is vital to all of our well being. Having liaised with thousands and worked with hundreds of people with 'mental illness' since 2002 and having been diagnosed with manic-depression myself in 1992 at the age of 17, I know that people lose their sanity for different reasons. It may be because of overwork, drugs, drink, relationship breakdown, other reasons or a combination of different reasons. People who experience 'mental illness', especially manic-depressive, always seem to get better if they can harness their creativity in some way or other.

I believe the same is true for every person. Everyone needs to harness their creativity in some way, shape or form, not just those who have a mental health related issue. They must have a creative outlet. If that creative outlet can be something that reminds them that their mad experiences can be used as a positive then that is where the real lasting change of well being can be possible. So write a book, do some art, create some music and send it in to the Chipmunkapublishing website. We are waiting to give you a voice, to encourage you to become a social entrepreneur to help others and the more you can promote yourself and believe in this mission, the more potential you will have to help others and the more we will be able to help you.

If you cannot see any kind of mental health related issue in your life or story then you are still welcome to send in your manuscript, music or art in. You may be surprised to discover that there is a mental health angle in everything.

If you are going to write a book and you do not know where to start then just think about your life for a moment. Since the age of 17 I have been absorbed in how the world perceives mental illness. When I was seventeen I was told I had manic-depression and that this was a disorder/disease that I would have for the rest of my life. Having written my own autobiography on living with manic-depression *A Can of Madness* and published nearly 250 books on mental illness in the last 5 years I now see that everyone's life is affected by mental illness. If I can make everyone in the world realise that they have an aspect of a mental health issue in their lives then Chipmunka as a publisher will have made the transition from Mental Health Survivor Publisher to Well Being Publisher. Therefore the perception will have changed. Instead of people self-manifesting their own mental illness and being stigmatised by people, the world will be more concerned with well being and improving each other's lives.

During my own recovery I have gone through different stages and controlled creativity has been present when I have made the quantum leap into well being. Below is my list of the titles of my first 5 books. I want you to come up with your 5 titles for your first 5 books. Even if you have never written a book or never envisaged writing a book, I want you to come up with 5 titles now so you can move your well being score up from 85% to 90%.

1) A Can of Madness
2) Curing Madness
3) The Ultimate Guide To Well Being
4) Mental Health Empowerment
5) Happiness in 7 Seconds

The Ultimate Guide to Well Being

Your 5 titles for your first 5 books

1)
2)
3)
4)
5)

We all are, or can be creative to a lesser or greater degree if we are given the opportunity. In the next few lines I will explain exactly what creativity is. Creativity always involves thinking or behaving imaginatively. Second, overall this imaginative activity is purposeful: that is, it is directed to achieving an objective. Third, these processes must generate something original. Fourth, the outcome must be of value in relation to the objective.

Creativity improves people's self-esteem, motivation and achievement.

People who are encouraged to think creatively and independently become:

   More interested in discovering things for themselves
   More open to new ideas
   Keen to work with others to explore ideas

Now we know what creativity is, let's have some fun with it. Now I want you to come up with 5 titles for recording your own music album. I'll help with coming up with titles of my own. My genre is rap. You can choose whatever musical genre you want?

1)   A Can of Madness
2)   Raps To Recovery
3)   The Maddest Rapper In The World
4)   Empowerment
5)   Mad Ghetto

List the 5 names of the albums you are thinking of recording:

1)

2)

3)

4)

5)

This brings your well being score up from 90% to 95% as long as you have put the title down for each album. If you actually go on to make the albums and they become successful, remember what inspired you to produce them and please

The Ultimate Guide to Well Being

make a donation to The Chipmunka Foundation
(registered charity number 1109537). All the
money will go towards helping people with mental
health issues. If you cannot find a record label or
do not want to set up your own website to sell it
then you know where to send them in, we are
waiting. Thank you for your kindness. Now one
last task for that maximum score.

Although I am a writer and have recorded a rap
album I am certainly not an artist. I am fortunate to
know one or two extremely talented artists. The
best advice one of them gave me when I asked
them how I should paint was – just paint. This is
what I say to people who want to write their own
book and also similar to what I was advised when
doing my rap album. Now I am going to challenge
you and myself to come up with 5 works of art.
You will see that there is already some excellent
art on the Chipmunkapublishing website.

Here are my 5 titles of art. Once I write them down
I commit to painting them before my fourth book
comes out.

1)   A Can of Madness –
2)   The Secret Art of A Manic-Depressive
3)   Mad Art
4)   From Madness to Well Being
5)   Empowering Mad Artists Around The World

Your top 5 art masterpieces will be:

1)
2)
3)
4)
5)

Congratulations you have now increased your score from 95% to 100 percent. You now have 100 percent well being.

Now how do you feel having written the 5 titles to your first 5 books? How do you feel? Pretty creative… Good. How do you feel knowing that writing those books could be used to reduce stigma on mental health and give a voice to people with mental illness, even better... Great… It's up to you if you want to write a book or not, but being creative is something that every human being should be encouraged to do. It is good for the human spirit and our sanity as long as we maintain our practical and logical side too.

There is of course more to creativity than writing, music and art but they are great examples, as each of these disciplines requires the use of different senses.

During your journey to 100% Ultimate Well being you have learnt to master many different positive states of well being. You have discovered how to measure having a healthy mind, body and soul. You have learnt what is crucial to your happiness. You have inspired yourself and become more aware of inspiring and having time for other people. You have worked on how to make the world a better place. You have connected with your spirituality and the spirituality of other people and rid yourself of your ego. You have mastered making the impossible possible by being aware of emotional intelligence and altering your perception. You have also harnessed your creativity.

Taking all this into consideration you deserve to have achieved 100% well being and there is no reason why you should not be able to maintain 100% Ultimate Well Being throughout your life. Before you sit back, relax and celebrate, spare a though for enabling other people you come into contact with in life achieving Ultimate Well Being as well. Not only is this a comforting thought but focusing on the happiness of others on a daily basis is also the key to your Ultimate Well Being. It's not rocket science, anyone can achieve it. I wish you 100% ultimate well being and the same for the people that you come into contact with. It has been a pleasure writing this book. If it has helped you in anyway, then I would love to hear about it. You can contact me through the publishing company's website at www.chipmunkapublishing.com or direct at

Jason Pegler

jasonpegler@chipmunkapublishing.com. Thanks
for listening. May the force of Ultimate Well Being
be with you always.

Conclusion

Ultimate Well Being Contract

I make a commitment to myself to snap out of any negative thoughts that may arise and focus on Ultimate Well Being for the rest of my life.

I make a full commitment to myself to have a Healthy Mind, Body and Soul

I know what is crucial to your happiness and will ensure that I use this knowledge to maintain my happiness.

I know how to inspire myself and will therefore be at ease inspiring myself every day.

I will Inspire and have time for other people at every reasonable opportunity.

I dedicate myself to making the world a better place?

I promise to connecting myself spiritually and to let go of my ego.

I endeavour to making the impossible possible by using emotional intelligence wherever possible.

Jason Pegler

I will harness my creativity to improve my well being and enable the well being of others.

I realise that signing this contract is a life long commitment to increasing my well being and that of other people.

signed by

_____

date